Food Safety and Quality Assurance

FOODS OF ANIMAL ORIGIN

Food Safety & Quality Assurance

FOODS OF ANIMAL ORIGIN

WILLIAM T. HUBBERT, D.V.M., M.P.H., Ph.D., Dipl. A.C.V.P.M.
Director, Residue Evaluation and Planning Division
Food Safety and Inspection Service
United States Department of Agriculture

HARRY V. HAGSTAD, D.V.M., M.P.H., Dipl. A.C.V.P.M., Fellow A.C.E.
Professor Emeritus, Department of Epidemiology and Community Health
School of Veterinary Medicine, Louisiana State University

WITH CONTRIBUTIONS BY

ELIZABETH SPANGLER, D.V.M., Ph.D., Dipl. A.C.V.P.M.
Atlantic Veterinary College
University of Prince Edward Island

IOWA STATE UNIVERSITY PRESS / AMES

♾ Printed on acid-free paper in the United States of America

First edition, 1991

Library of Congress Cataloging-in-Publication Data
Hubbert, William T.
    Food safety & quality assurance: foods of animal origin / William T. Hubbert, Harry V. Hagstad: with contributions by Elizabeth Spangler.—1st ed.
        p.   cm.
    Based on Food quality control: a syllabus for veterinary students, published in 1982, and Food quality control: foods of animal origin, published in 1986, both by Harry V. Hagstad and William T. Hubbert.
    Includes bibliographical references and index.
    ISBN 0-8138-0708-5
    1. Animal food—Health aspects. 2. Animal food—Contamination. 3. Food industry and trade—Quality control. 4. Foodborne diseases—Prevention. 5. Food adulteration and inspection. I. Hagstad, Harry V. II. Spangler, Elizabeth. III. Hagstad, Harry V. Food quality control. IV. Title. V. Title: Food safety and quality assurance.
RA601.H62 1991
664′.907—dc20   91-11818

CONTENTS

PREFACE

This text is an outgrowth of *Food Quality Control: A Syllabus for Veterinary Students,* which was published in 1982, and *Food Quality Control: Foods of Animal Origin,* which was published in 1986. Overall, this edition is approximately 20 percent larger than the previous edition. Major additions include production of ducks and rabbits in Chapter 1, and hazard analysis critical control points, as well as inspection, in Canada in Chapter 3. Because of the rapid changes in aquatic animal production worldwide, that section has undergone considerable revision. Similarly, the section on controlling chemical adulteration has been revised in accordance with increasing public and governmental concern. This edition includes new figures and tables, as well as updates of those from earlier editions. Throughout the text, comments from the review panel have been particularly valuable in identifying areas in need of addition or revision.

Unlike texts in which attention is focused on only one segment of food animal production or processing, in *Food Safety and Quality Assurance* an overall view of the food chain is presented so that the reader may better recognize potential sources of contamination.

The purpose of this text is to prepare students to

1. Identify human health hazards in foods of animal origin
2. Identify the role of veterinarians in preventing introduction of hazards into the food chain
3. Identify agencies and their activities in regard to maintaining safety and wholesomeness of foods of animal origin
4. Identify principles of safe food handling and processing
5. Collect and analyze data relevant to investigation of foodborne disease outbreaks

The *Task Analysis and Curriculum Planning Guide* (1981), developed by the Conference of Teachers of Food Hygiene and published by the U.S. Department of Agriculture, Denton, Texas, served as the principal guide for topics presented in the first edition. Material presented in the descriptions of microbial and nonmicrobial contaminants and the section on consumer protection is designed to serve as a guide to current knowledge and regulations. In-depth information may be obtained from the standard texts and publications listed in the bibliographies following each chapter.

ACKNOWLEDGMENTS

The authors are deeply indebted to the following persons who constituted a review panel to evaluate the second edition of this text. Their comments and suggestions were invaluable in the development of this edition.

Dr. A. Atkinson
Tuskegee University
Tuskegee, Alabama

Dr. Asa B. Childers
Texas A&M University
College Station, Texas

Dr. David W. Dreesen
University of Georgia
Athens, Georgia

Dr. Constantin Genigeorgis
University of California
Davis, California

Dr. John C. Gordon
Ohio State University
Columbus, Ohio

Dr. Charles S. McCain
Oklahoma State University
Stillwater, Oklahoma

Dr. Gilles Morin
University of Montreal
Quebec, Canada

Dr. David A.A. Mossel
University of Utrecht
Utrecht, Netherlands

Dr. Kevin D. Pelzer
Virginia Polytechnic Institute
and State University
Blacksburg, Virginia

Dr. P. Seneviratna
Murdoch University
Murdoch, Western Australia

Dr. Richard E. Smith
Louisiana State University
Baton Rouge, Louisiana

Dr. Ronald D. Smith
University of Illinois
Urbana, Illinois

Dr. Elizabeth Spangler
Atlantic Veterinary College
Prince Edward Island, Canada

The authors wish to thank Drs. Tom Dukes, Wendell Grasse, Bob Macgregor, Doug Schurmann, and Craig Bellamy and Mr. Charles Cooke for help in preparing the section on inspection in Canada.

Food Safety and Quality Assurance

FOODS OF ANIMAL ORIGIN

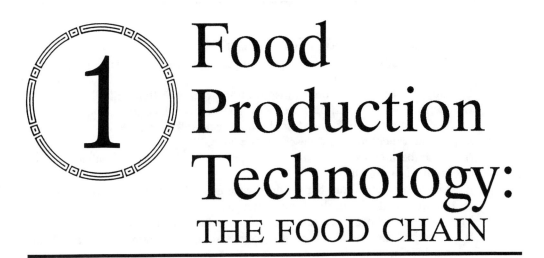

1 Food Production Technology:
THE FOOD CHAIN

A. PRODUCTION

Objectives

1. Livestock and Poultry Producers and Areas
   a) Distinguish between subsistence agriculture and commercial agriculture and indicate ways in which the differences affect veterinary medicine.
   b) Identify the major geographic areas in the world associated with production of the following: livestock grazing or ranching, intensive cattle management systems, sheep and goats, swine, poultry (chickens, ducks, turkeys), and rabbits.
   c) Distinguish between noncompetitive and competitive agricultural imports and indicate an influence that veterinary medicine may have on the quantity of competitive products imported.
   d) Briefly describe the general demographic characteristics of the United States farm population (human) as a prototype client of a food-animal practitioner.
   e) Describe the major types of tenure among producer enterprises in relation to geographic trends related to type of livestock and poultry production.
   f) Identify areas within the United States with concentrations of the following specific types of animal production: beef cows and feedlots; dairy farms; general livestock farms; and production of sheep, swine, broilers, turkeys, eggs, ducks, horses, goats, and rabbits.

2. Milk Production
   a) Identify the factors that influence production and consumption of various dairy products in the United States.

b) Define milkshed.

c) Explain how the price of milk is established.

d) Differentiate between necessary surplus, constant surplus, and seasonal surplus.

e) Describe the storage and transportation process of fluid milk.

f) Define the goals and purpose of an abnormal-milk control program.

g) Define mastitic milk and describe how such milk is detected.

h) Define rancid milk and describe its causes.

i) Describe how to investigate a herd problem associated with high bacterial counts in the milk.

j) List recommendations to prevent environmental contamination from creating an abnormal-milk problem on the farm.

k) Describe the two basic functions of a milking machine system.

l) Describe the functions of the four essential components of a milking machine system.

m) Describe important design and functional characteristics of the vacuum- and milk-line systems in a milking operation.

n) Describe the action within the teat cup during the milking sequence that indicates pressure changes as they occur to draw the milk from the udder to the line.

o) Describe the function and operation of the pulsator.

3. Aquatic Animal Production
   a) Vertebrate fish production
      1) Explain the importance of marine fish species in terms of world food supplies.
      2) Describe catfish farming and associated health-related management problems.
      3) Describe sanitation problems associated with techniques of harvesting marine fish.
   b) Shellfish production
      1) Indicate the categories of commercially important shellfish.
      2) Describe shellfish harvesting and its relation to the production of wholesome products.
      3) Describe restrictions on shellfish harvesting that involve environmental contamination.

Text

1. Livestock and Poultry Producers and Areas

a) *Classification of economic activities.* Although in a classic sense veterinary medicine is concerned with health maintenance in animal populations, veterinarians must deal with human clients (either private or public) to accomplish their goals. Therefore, the practice of veterinary medicine affects the two production aspects of economic activity: (1) primarily by increasing the harvest of animal agriculture, and (2) secondarily by increasing the value of foods of animal origin as a result of food safety and quality assurance.

1) *Subsistence agriculture.* In a subsistence economy, there is little or no

surplus to be offered for sale. Because cash is not generated to pay for the service of a veterinarian, most veterinarians are employed by public agencies.

(a) *Subsistence farming.* In large areas of the world, primitive subsistence farming prevails.

(b) *Subsistence herding.* In still other large areas, subsistence herding is the predominant agricultural activity. Frequently, animal diseases are a major factor in limiting production from such herding to the subsistence level. Infection and undernutrition (mismanagement) reduce the quantity and quality of animal units produced. Also, infections transmitted between animals and humans (such as brucellosis and tuberculosis) are often prevalent in the human population and reduce the efficiency of human labor.

2) *Percentage of active population employed in primary sector.* In the areas where subsistence farming or herding predominate, usually more than 75 percent of the active population (work force) is employed in the primary sector (mainly agriculture).

b) *Livestock production areas.* Livestock production can be classified regionally according to the principal species or types of livestock produced.

1) *Undeveloped areas.* In some areas, such as the central regions of Africa, Australia, and South America, there is practically no livestock. In these areas, hunting and fishing provide most of the animal protein consumed.

2) *Livestock ranching worldwide.* The major livestock ranching areas of the world are those where sheep, cattle, and goats are grazed principally to produce wool, hides, or meat. In some areas (such as the western United States), animals are sold for meat or to others who fatten them before slaughter. The United States ranks among the leading livestock-raising countries in all species except goats. Much of the goat population in the leading goat-producing nations is of the Angora type (used to produce mohair) rather than the milking breeds.

3) *Intensive livestock management areas*

(a) *Cattle production worldwide.* Three areas of dense commercial cattle population exist: the midwestern United States, central Europe, and the east coast of South America.

(b) *Dairy farming worldwide.* On a worldwide basis, centers for commercial milk production are limited to certain portions of the United States, north-central Europe, the southeastern coast of Australia, and the north island of New Zealand. There are two main reasons for these limitations: (1) a large part of the world does not drink milk, and (2) the areas where milk is not an important dietary item also lack the technology of handling milk in fluid form or producing a stable powder. A large part of the production in Australia and New Zealand is used to produce a high-quality milk powder for export. Since a large percentage of the milk produced is used to manufacture powder for export, the dairy industry makes maximum use of the seasonal fluctuations in pasture growth. Calving is timed to coincide with the onset of increasing growth (early spring), and cows are dry during the period of least growth (late winter). Particularly, in New Zealand, hilly terrain and high fertilizer costs restrict the production and feeding of concentrates. Therefore, milk yields represent essentially the potential from dairy cows on a grass diet.

(c) *Sheep production worldwide*. The interior of Australia is the foremost sheep-producing area of the world. Australian sheep have been selected to produce the world's finest-quality wool for garment cloth. Other areas produce wools of lesser grade (such as carpet wools) or raise meat breeds primarily. New Zealand, for example, ships large quantities of lamb to England and other foreign markets. The emphasis on export is clear from the local term for abattoirs as "freezer works."

(d) *Swine production worldwide*. The three centers for swine production in the world are the upper midwestern United States, central Europe, and China.

(e) *Poultry production worldwide*. China, the United States, and the USSR are the world leaders in poultry production. In 1988, estimated total numbers (in millions) of poultry stock worldwide and leading countries were as follows (*FAO Production Yearbook*, 1988):

Chickens		Ducks		Turkeys	
World	10,215	World	519	World	223
China	1,849	China	325	USA	78
USA	1,540	Bangladesh	32	USSR	48
USSR	1,129	Indonesia	29	Italy	23
Brazil	550	Viet Nam	27	France	20
Indonesia	410	Thailand	16	Mexico	12
Japan	334	France	11	UK	9
India	260	Mexico	7	Israel	7
Mexico	224	USA	7	Canada	6

(f) *Rabbit production worldwide*. Although solid statistics on domestic rabbit production are scarce, France is probably the leading producer. Other countries with recognized industries include Belgium, Germany, Italy, USSR, Scandinavia, Switzerland, China, India, United States, and United Kingdom. In addition to meat, skins and angora wool are significant sources of income.

c) *Imports*

1) *Noncompetitive (complimentary) agricultural imports*. The United States imports large quantities of noncompetitive agricultural products that are not produced domestically. These include such commodities as coffee, cocoa, natural rubber, bananas, tea, spices, and carpet wool. (See Fig. 1.1.)

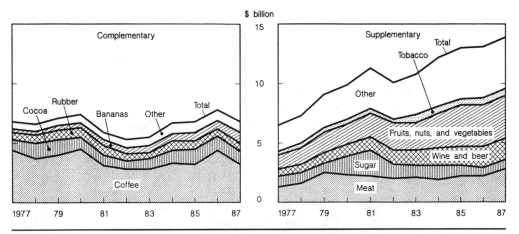

Fig. 1.1. U.S. agricultural imports by commodity, 1977–1987. Complementary imports are those that do not compete with U.S. agricultural products, such as coffee, cocoa, and bananas. Supplementary imports compete with domestically produced products such as meat and sugar.

2) *Competitive (supplementary) imports.* In addition, the United States imports large quantities of products that are also produced in the United States. These include meats, sugar and molasses, fruits and vegetables, wine, oilseeds, and dairy products and eggs, as well as cattle and calves. Beef represents approximately 80 percent of the red meat imported. These foreign products compete in the U.S. domestic market. At present, there are import limitations on the quantities of meat and some other products of animal origin. First, the government has established quotas by country on the amount of meat that may be imported. Second, countries in which foot-and-mouth disease is endemic cannot export any fresh meat into the United States (*cooked* meat can be imported). Some large exporters of fresh meat such as Argentina are thus excluded from our market. If foot-and-mouth disease is eradicated from these areas, serious pressure on the U.S. domestic market may come from these foreign sources. Residues of antibiotics, sulfonamides, and other chemicals are becoming an additional important issue for U.S. exports, particularly to Japan and the European Economic Community (EEC).

3) *Meat exporters to the United States.* In fiscal year (FY) 1988, the five leading exporters of beef and veal to the United States (in decreasing order by product weight) were Australia, New Zealand, Canada, Argentina, and Brazil. New Zealand and Australia were the only significant exporters of lamb and mutton. Canada, Denmark, Sweden, and Finland were the four significant exporters of pork. Note that Argentina and Brazil are major exporters of beef and veal in spite of the requirement that all their products must be cooked. This is true as well for pork from Sweden and Finland.

d) *Demography of the U.S. farm population*
  1) *Farm population*. In the United States, the farm population has been decreasing at a steady rate. The farm population is now less than 10 percent of the total in most states. Even in a state such as Iowa, where agriculture is the leading business, less than 20 percent actually live on farms. (See Fig. 1.2.)
  2) *Farms*. Nationwide, the number of farms is decreasing. Although some land has been shifted from agriculture to other uses, the primary reason for the decrease in farm numbers is that the average size of farms is increasing. Fewer farmers are managing larger acreage. The average size of farms generally increases from east to west, which is partly a reflection of productivity per acre.
  3) *Agriculture and urbanization in the United States*. Since the turn of the century, the United States population has been moving from the farm to urban areas. Even among the rural population, there is a shift from strictly agricultural employment to nonagricultural pursuits, which include services to agriculture such as those performed by veterinarians. The greatest shift from the farm has occurred in the South.
  4) *Sex ratio of the U.S. population by age*. A comparison of the sex ratio of the rural farm population by age group (number of males per 100 females) with the rural nonfarm and urban populations reveals that the farm population is predominantly older males. This means in general that veterinarians will be dealing with older men (and their long-standing opinions and methods) as part of food animal practice. Young people have left the farm for greater opportunities in the city.
e) *Tenure*
  1) *Land in farms by tenure of operator*. The farm manager may own the farm outright, have one or more partners, or rent the land. Larger farms

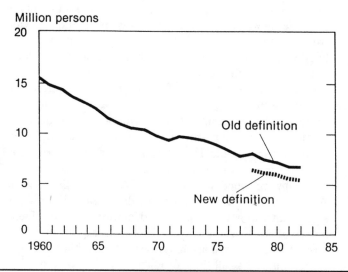

Fig. 1.2. Farm population in the United States, 1960–1985. (Census Bureau)

(those in the West) are less likely to be owned by individuals. Similarly, larger farms are more likely to be operated by partnership.

2) *Land in farms operated by corporations.* The largest farms are generally operated by corporations. In contrast to subsistence farmers, large operators tend to have capital and qualified managers and thus employ veterinarians in developing efficient herd health programs.

3) *Farms operated by tenants.* The frequency of tenant operations also is somewhat higher in the west. In many instances, these may be large tracts that are leased for agricultural purposes rather than those operated by small tenant farmers.

4) *Farms operated by full owners.* Although nationwide, most farms are operated (managed) by the owners, there are some differences among livestock enterprises. Generally, a greater percentage of dairy farm operators own their own enterprises, compared with other livestock operations, which tend to be run by managers.

f) *Animal production areas in the United States.*

1) *Beef cows, feedlots, and livestock farms.* Although the total number of cattle has increased in the United States during the past 20 yr, the number of dairy cattle has decreased significantly. Therefore, beef cattle are responsible for the growth in population. General livestock farms are most numerous in the Midwest, with the greatest concentration in Iowa. (See Fig. 1.3.)

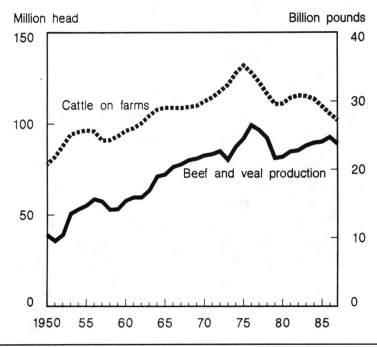

Fig. 1.3. Cattle numbers and beef production in the United States, 1945-1985. (USDA)

(a) *Pastureland as a percentage of land in farms.* Progressing from east to west, there is a steady increase in percentage of farmland used for pasture, from considerably less than 50 percent to more than 75 percent.

(b) *Cattle and calves: Increase and decrease.* There has been a decrease in numbers of cattle in the eastern United States during the past few years with a corresponding increase in the large feedlot centers in the Texas panhandle, Imperial valley of California, and Gila valley of Arizona. Many of the cattle in the Midwest, however, are fattened in much smaller numbers on general farms.

(c) *Feedlot size.* As one would expect, the increase in number of feedlot-fattened cattle has been related not only to a greater number of feedlot operations but to a growth in capacity of existing feedlots. Many of the larger operations can handle 50,000-100,000 head at a time. (See Fig. 1.4.)

(d) *Meat-packing: Cattle.* The concentrations of abattoirs slaughtering large numbers of cattle are associated geographically with the principal areas where cattle are fattened. Some abattoirs, however, are located near large population centers because of (1) a nearby market for fresh meat and (2) slaughter of cull dairy cattle from dairies in large milksheds supplying these urban areas.

2) *Dairy farms*

(a) *Location.* The greatest number of dairy farms in the United States

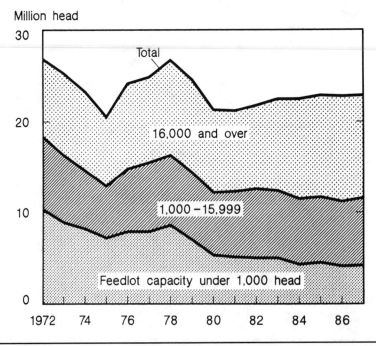

Fig. 1.4. Fed cattle marketed in the United States, by feedlot capacity, 1945–1985. (USDA)

are in Wisconsin and Minnesota. Although these states have many dairy farms, the number of cows per farm is relatively small. Much of this milk is used to produce manufactured dairy products, such as cheese. On the other hand, larger concentrations of dairy cattle tend to be close to large population centers to supply fluid milk. (See Fig. 1.5.) In northeastern United States, Alaska, the island of Oahu in Hawaii, southern California (except the Imperial valley), and the areas adjacent to Miami, the cattle raised are almost exclusively dairy cattle.

(b) *Milk cows: Increase and decrease.* During the past few years, there has been a significant decrease nationwide in the number of dairy cows. This is an indication of the economic problems currently affecting the dairy industry. Although the ratio of milk cows to replacement stock has remained relatively constant, the total numbers of both have decreased steadily.

(c) *Milk production.* The total milk production in the United States has remained relatively constant during the past several years. This is the result of an increase in production per cow sufficient to counteract a decrease in number of cows. Dairy herd improvement records for 1988 indicate that cows representing the five major dairy breeds produced (on the basis of a 305-day lactation period and milking 2 × per day) between 11,890 and 17,275 lb (5405 and 7852

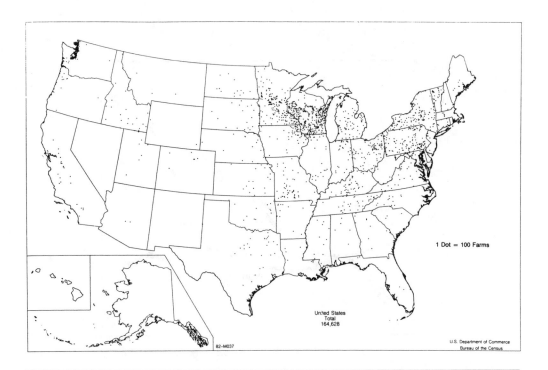

Fig. 1.5. Dairy farms in the United States, 1982. (Census Bureau)

kg) of milk with a fat percentage between 3.7 and 4.8 percent. Considering 1 gal of milk to weigh 8.3 lb, the average dairy cow produced between 4.7 and 6.8 gal (17.8 and 25.7 l) per day during a 10-mo lactation period (See Fig. 1.6.). The average milk production per cow increased by one-third during the 5-yr period 1983–1988. Much of this increase resulted from extensive culling of less productive animals. With the advent of bovine somatotropin (BST), another jump in per cow production is possible. It is unlikely, however, that BST-enhanced milk production will become a common practice until widespread concerns of consumers are dealt with.

3) *Sheep and lambs.* Central Texas is the leading area in the United States in sheep production, with the Sacramento valley of California second. Sheep are raised in moderate numbers throughout the remainder of the United States except for the Southeast, where parasites and humidity have combined to discourage commercial sheep production. Since the beginning of World War II, sheep production in the United States has been declining. The demand for wool has decreased because of the widespread use of synthetic fibers. In addition, lamb has never been a favorite in the average American diet. (See Fig. 1.7.)

4) *Swine.* Swine production in the United States is centered in Iowa. A secondary producing area extends along the eastern coastal plain from Maryland to southeastern Alabama. Recently, the center of swine production has had a southerly shift in the Midwest and a significant

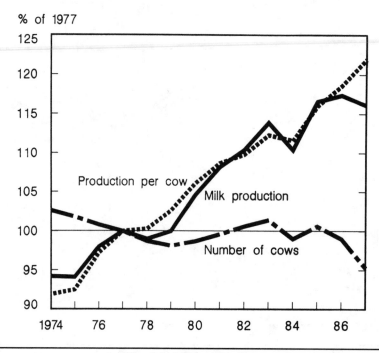

Fig. 1.6. Milk production, number of cows, and milk per cow in the United States, 1974–1986.

increase along the East Coast. The abattoirs in the United States that slaughter hogs are located primarily in association with the swine-producing areas. (See Fig. 1.8.)

5) *Poultry*

(a) *Chickens*. Broiler farms are concentrated in Georgia, Alabama, and Arkansas. The distribution of laying hens is related to the market for fresh eggs in large urban centers nearby. Significant numbers of laying hens in some areas are producing eggs to hatch out chicks for broiler production. (See Fig. 1.9.)

(b) *Ducks*. Commercial duck production is concentrated in the 12 states where the 29 federally inspected abattoirs are located. New York, California, Indiana, and Wisconsin are the leading producing states.

(c) *Turkeys*. Turkeys are raised for meat in large numbers in the states from Minnesota to Texas. Much of the hatching of turkey poults for these rearing operations is done in California. (See Fig. 1.10.)

6) *Horses and ponies*. Interestingly, the horse population has a very even distribution nationwide except for a concentration in a small area near Lexington, Kentucky (Fig. 1.11). Although most of the more than 8 million horses in the United States are used for pleasure riding and racing, some are slaughtered for human consumption. There are 17 federally inspected abattoirs in 7 states. In fiscal year 1987, more than 276,000 horses were inspected, slightly less than the more than 300,000 inspected annually in the late 1970s. Much of the horsemeat, more than 63 million lb (28.5 million kg) produced in FY 1983 was exported. More than half was shipped to France.

7) *Goats*. Goats are of minor economic significance in the United States. The largest population (Angoras) is located in Texas. Dairy herd improvement records for dairy goats were first published in 1968, an indication of the recent increase in the size of the U.S. national herd. In 1988, goats representing all major dairy breeds produced an average of 1816 lb (825 kg) of milk with 3.76 percent fat.

8) *Rabbits*. Rabbits are produced in small backyard rabbitries throughout the United States with their greatest popularity probably in California. Federal inspection of rabbits at slaughter for meat is a voluntary program and only two plants, one in Arkansas and one in North Carolina, participate.

2. Milk Production

a) *U.S. dairy industry*. The dairy industry is one of the largest food industries in the United States, with dairy products contributing 16 percent to the gross national product (GNP) of the food industry. Consumers spend more than $12 billion annually for dairy products, approximately 60 percent of which is spent for fluid milk and cream. Approximately 47–50 percent of the milk produced each year is consumed as fluid milk and cream, nearly 20 percent is used to manufacture butter, 16–20 percent for cheese, 9–10 percent for ice cream and 3–4 percent for evaporated and condensed milk; the remainder is used in other ways, such as feeding animals. Nationwide, dairying earns about 12 percent of the cash farm income, whereas in Wisconsin, the leading

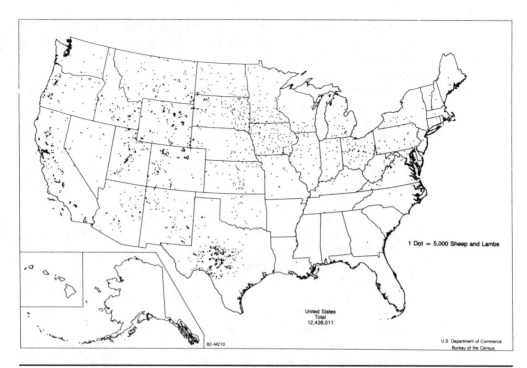

Fig. 1.7.   Sheep and lambs in the United States, 1982.
(Census Bureau)

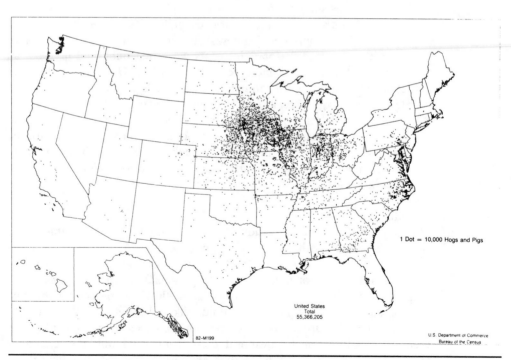

Fig. 1.8.   Hogs and pigs in the United States, 1982. (Census
Bureau)

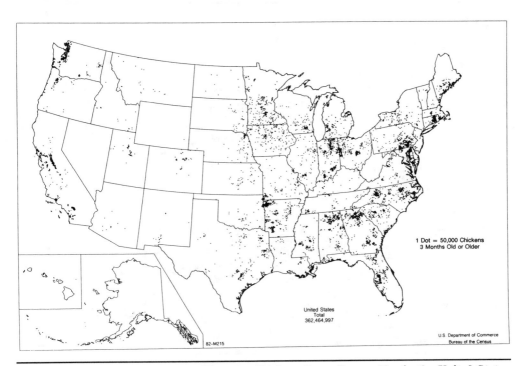

Fig. 1.9. Chickens 3 months or older in the United States, 1982. (Census Bureau)

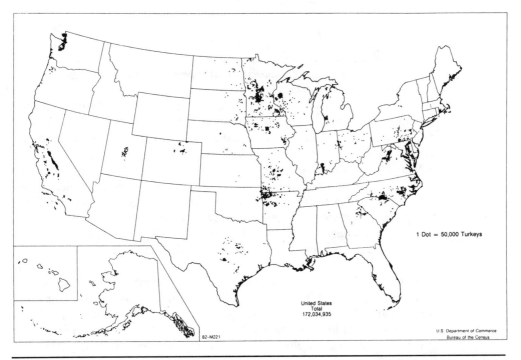

Fig. 1.10. Turkeys sold in the United States, 1982. (Census Bureau)

15

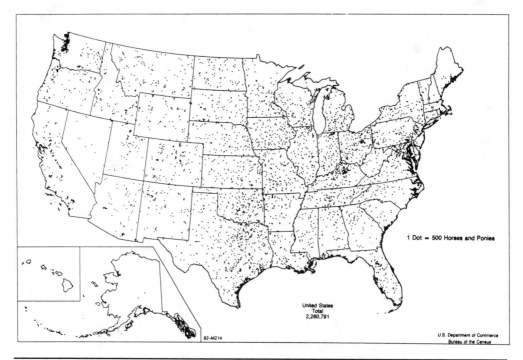

Fig. 1.11. Horses and ponies in the United States, 1982. (Census Bureau)

dairy state, it represents more than one-half the cash farm income. The centers for producing manufactured products from milk are mainly in the northern and northeastern states, where several factors combine to permit economical milk production.

b) *Milksheds*. Just as the water in a river comes from a well-defined watershed, the milk supply to a municipality comes from a well-defined *milkshed*, or producing area. The size of the milkshed depends largely on the size of the consuming population. The size of the producing farm (i.e., the number of milking cows per herd) determines the area needed in the milkshed to serve a given consumer population. In the United States, there is a trend toward larger dairy herds from north to south. Among herds participating in the Dairy Herd Improvement Association (DHIA) program in 1988, the average number of cows per herd was smallest in Alaska (63) and largest in Arizona (590). Some herds supplying the Miami milkshed maintain more than 5000 cows.

c) *Milk pricing.* Most of the milk produced in the United States is marketed by dairy cooperatives, which may be either fluid milk associations or dairy product manufacturing and marketing associations. The farmer is paid on a unit base of 100 lb, (11.6 gal, 45.4 kg, or 43.8 l) fluid milk produced. The consumer price index (all items) is one component of a formula often used to compute prices.

d) *Seasonal variation in milk supply*. Each milkshed must maintain an adequate milk supply to be sure that in periods of low milk production there is enough milk to meet the demand for fluid milk. To do this, a large supply of milk is maintained in periods of peak production so the demand can be met when production is low. The quantity of milk utilized for fluid sales is fairly uniform throughout the year. A *necessary surplus* is needed to offset daily fluctuations in demand and is used in the manufacture of Grade A dairy products such as cottage cheese. A *constant surplus* is available even during periods of lowest production should an unexpected decrease in production (e.g., from shortage of pasture) or increase in demand occur. A constant surplus that is greater than needed is a major indicator of overproduction in the milkshed and a major cause of lowered prices paid to the producer. A *seasonal surplus* occurs when seasonal patterns of breeding result in seasonal peaks in freshening and correspondingly higher production early in the lactation cycle. The seasonal surplus may be handled in a surplus-processing plant that processes fluid milk into manufactured products that can be stored and used later. (See Fig. 1.12.)

e) *Milk storage and transport.* Milk is stored on the farm and transported to the receiving station or plant in one of two ways: the can system or the bulk tank system.

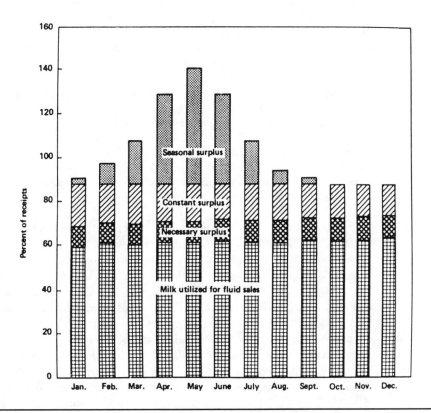

Fig. 1.12. Seasonal variations in milk supply in the United States. The kinds of milk surplus are (1) necessary or stand-by, (2) constant, and (3) seasonal.

1) *Can system.* Tinned metal, aluminum, or stainless steel cans, usually of 37.8-l (10-gal) capacity, are sometimes used to store milk on the farm. The cans are cooled on the farm in tanks of refrigerated water or in cabinet coolers using a cold water spray.

2) *Bulk tank system.* Today milk is handled almost exclusively in bulk containers beginning with a mechanically refrigerated stainless steel bulk tank for storage in the farm milk house. Milk in this tank is cooled rapidly by contact with a refrigerated expansion plate that is an integral part of the inner liner at the bottom of the tank. Another type of bulk tank uses an ice water spray on the sides of the inner shell of the tank to cool the milk.

3) *Transport.* Tank trucks pick up the milk from the farm and deliver it to the receiving station or dairy plant. At a receiving station, the milk is cooled, weighed, pooled, and stored until it is shipped to a large dairy plant in trucks or railroad cars. The receiving station must be equipped to sample and test milk as well as to clean tank trucks.

f) *Abnormal-milk control program.* In 1967, the Food and Drug Administration of the U.S. Public Health Service (FDA/USPHS) initiated an abnormal-milk control program. The two main goals of the program are (1) *education* of the industry regarding the effect of mastitis on milk quality nationwide and (2) *regulation* of the industry in order to fulfill the consumer's expectation of a clean, safe, wholesome product derived from healthy cows. The program is to develop a proper and uniform interpretation of the Grade A Pasteurized Milk Ordinance that defines *abnormal milk* as follows:

> Cows which show evidence of the secretion of abnormal milk in one or more quarters, based upon bacteriologic, chemical or physical examination shall be milked last or with separate equipment; and the milk shall be *discarded*. Cows treated with, or cows which have consumed chemical, medicinal, or radioactive agents which are capable of being secreted in the milk and which, in the judgment of the health authority, may be deleterious to human health, shall be milked last or with separate equipment, and the milk disposed of as the health authority may direct.

g) *Mastitic milk. Mastitic milk* is defined as milk containing excessive numbers of somatic cells. Normal milk seldom has more than 1,000,000 cells/ml.

1) *Screening tests for mastitic milk.* Four tests used commonly for screening raw milk samples for somatic cell levels are: the California Mastitis Test (CMT), Wisconsin Mastitis Test (WMT), Modified Whiteside Test (MWT), and Catalase Test (CT). In three instances, the test is based on cell viscosity; the CMT also includes pH change. The fourth test measures release of the intracellular enzyme catalase. (See Table 1.1.)

2) *Confirmatory tests for mastitic milk.* If the screening test is positive, a *confirmatory cell count* is required using either a direct microscopic or an electronic counting technique. If the confirmatory count exceeds 1,500,000 cells/ml, the producer is sent a notice listing the more likely causes. If two of the last four consecutive counts exceed 1,500,000 cells, an inspection is performed at milking time. If three of the last five

Table 1.1. Interpretation of screening tests for abnormal milk

Test	Score or Reading	Somatic Cells (Leukocytes/ml Milk
California Mastitis Test (CMT)	N	0–200,000
	T	150,000–500,000
	1	400,000–1,500,000
	2	800,000–5,000,000
	3	>5,000,000
Modified Whiteside Test (MWT)	N	<500,000
	T	500,000–1,000,000
	1+	1,000,000–2,000,000
	2+	1,500,000–3,000,000
	3+	>3,000,000
Wisconsin Mastitis Test (WMT)	<10mm	<500,000
	10–20mm	500,000–900,000
	>20mm	>1,000,000
Catalase Test (CT)	<20%	<500,000
	20–30%	500,000–1,000,000
	30–40%	1,000,000–2,000,000
	>40%	>2,000,000

Note: N = negative, T = trace.

counts exceed 1,500,000 cells, the producer's permit is suspended. The producer must submit a written statement indicating that the causes have been corrected, followed by a satisfactory inspection and sample test, before reinstatement.

h) *Rancidity.* *Rancidity* is the presence in milk of an undesirable flavor caused by certain free fatty acids. Only a small amount of normal milk fat needs to be split by the enzyme lipase to glycerol and fatty acids to cause rancid flavor. Rancidity is of two types, *induced* and *spontaneous*. If the flavor is present in freshly drawn milk, it is not rancidity.

1) *Induced rancidity.* Induced rancidity results when the lipase normally present in raw milk is activated. Three principal causes of lipase activation are (1) agitation or foaming (prolonged shaking of warm raw milk), (2) temperature fluctuations (warming precooled raw milk to about 30.5°C (87°F) and cooling it again, and (3) homogenization of raw milk or mixing raw milk with homogenized milk.

2) *Spontaneous rancidity.* Some cows produce milk that becomes rancid spontaneously when cooled and aged *without* activation. Spontaneous rancidity on a herd basis is most often seasonal, associated with the feeding of low-quality forage. When individual cows or herds are involved, the problem can be eliminated if potentially rancid milk is combined with 4 volumes of normal milk.

i) *Procedures when high bacterial count is reported.* Whenever a client's milk supply is reported to have a high bacterial count, the cause usually can be found with a little effort. The test must always be *repeated* to verify the count before panicking!

1) *Raw and pasteurized count comparison.* Comparison of raw and laborato-

ry pasteurized counts will give some clues as to the likely source of the problem. High raw and low pasteurized counts indicate contamination from cow or humans, whereas high raw and high pasteurized counts indicate environmental sources. If inadequate cooling is suspected, the cooling chart on the milk tank should be checked. If poor equipment cleaning seems likely, routine replacement of the teat cup liners is indicated; two sets of liners and other rubberware should be used, alternating them weekly to allow one to be cleaned and stored. High bacterial counts from poorly cleaned equipment indicate either contamination is building up at some point on the milk-handling surface or outside contamination from air lines, water, dust, etc.

2) *Sample collection and analysis.* If the problem persists, milk samples are collected for bacteriologic analysis at the end of each pipeline at the beginning, middle, and end of the milking period. The test results of these specimens in that area are analyzed to determine the needed corrective measures. In some instances, a further breakdown of samples may be needed, such as individual cow or milking unit samples, to pin point the source.

j) *Environmental contamination*

1) *Water.* The quality of water used on the farm is important for several reasons. Water may be a hazard to humans or animals on the farm if it is contaminated with pathogenic microorganisms. The USPHS Milk Ordinance of 1978 specifies that the water for milk house and milking operations shall be from a supply that is properly located, protected, and operated and should be easily accessible, adequate, and of a safe, sanitary quality. In hard-water areas, a film or scale (milkstone) collects on milk utensils (including rubberware) after they have been in use for some time as a result of interaction among milk solids, detergent, and hard water. Wherever this scale is deposited in the milking system, it is a potential habitat for microbial replication and high bacterial counts in milk. A mild organic acid such as phosphoric acid will remove the deposits.

2) *Pavement.* All areas subject to routine cow traffic should be paved for ease of general sanitation with a design that permits straight-line movement of mechanical cleaning equipment (e.g., skip loaders).

3) *Milking pit.* Whenever construction of a milk house, milking barn, or other building for a dairy is anticipated, health code requirements should be reviewed carefully during planning. In addition, the type of stall arrangement (gate, walk-through, or herringbone) to be used in the milking parlor should be considered in detail to determine the design that best meets individual needs. Such factors as herd size, number, competence of available milking machine operators, and climate will influence the decision. A poor choice creates management problems that will result in reduced production and quality of milk.

4) *Equipment cleaning.* Equipment cleaning consists of four separate steps: rinse, wash, rinse, and sanitize. The first rinse should be done as soon as possible (before the milk film dries) with a large volume of lukewarm water (hot water causes milkstone formation). Next, the equipment is

washed with an approved detergent at the appropriate concentration and length of time for adequate cleaning of the particular equipment (these factors may vary). To reduce milkstone, an organic acid detergent may be used at weekly intervals or an acidified rinse may be used routinely. The equipment must be rinsed thoroughly to remove the detergent solution. An approved chemical sanitizer is applied when the equipment is completely clean; otherwise its bactericidal activity is reduced by any residual cleaning compound or organic matter. Each component of the milking system has specific cleaning requirements. Some parts must be disassembled completely and cleaned by circulation or clean-in-place (CIP) methods. The vacuum line, although it does not transport milk, should be cleaned periodically for greatest efficiency. Health code requirements and manufacturers' recommendations should be guides for cleaning.

k) *Two requisites for conventional mechanical milking.* The milking machine performs two basic functions: (1) it imposes a controlled vacuum on the end of the teat to open the teat orifice and provide the differential pressure (suction) needed for milk flow, and (2) it massages the teat intermittently to continue stimulation and prevent blood congestion in the teat end. These two functions must be performed by a properly designed and comfortable liner (inflation). A poorly fitted liner may impair letdown or place undue stress on the teat and udder tissue. Vacuum fluctuations or improper massage may lead to mastitis by irritating the sensitive tissue of the teat canal.

l) *Four essential components of a milking machine system.*
(See Fig. 1.13.)

1) *Milking unit.* This is the part of the machine that is suspended from the cow, performs the milking operation, and receives the milk into a sanitary system. It includes the teat-cup assemblies, claw or suspension cup manifold and reservoir, and the connecting air and milk tubes.

2) *Pulsator.* This device controls the liner action by introducing vacuum and atmospheric pressure intermittently into the chamber between the liner and the teat-cup shell.

3) *Vacuum pump.* This pump provides a source of vacuum to the end of the teat to cause milk flow, supplies the energy to activate the liner and massage the teat, and moves the milk through the system.

4) *Receptacle.* The milk receptacle includes all hoses, pipes, and containers for conveying and holding the product. Systems are of two basic types: (1) a *bucket* system in which milk is received directly into a nearby vacuumized portable bucket and (2) a *pipeline* system that uses rigid stainless steel or heat-resistant-glass sanitary pipe for carrying vacuum from the milk receiver to the individual milking units and for carrying milk from the units to the milk receiver. In many areas, bucket systems have been replaced by pipelines because of greater labor efficiency.

m) *Vacuum and milk line system.*

1) *Vacuum lines.* The vacuum-supply piping connects the vacuum pump, reserve tank, sanitary trap just ahead of the milk receiver, and pulsator pipeline. An adequate pump is of no value if there is inadequate piping.

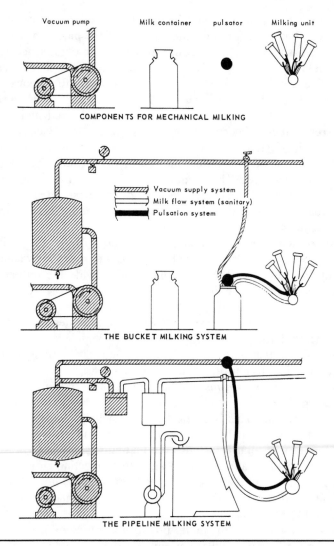

Fig. 1.13. **The four components of mechanical milking.**

2) *Milk lines*. The *milk line* conveys milk and air from the milking units to the receiver jar where the air is removed. Milk lines commonly installed are stainless steel tubing 2 in. (50.8 mm) or more in diameter. Most pipeline installations are now welded on the job into major assemblies. Welded milk lines look clean, improve sanitation, and prevent problems related to air leak, gaskets, and turbulence associated with union-type connections. All welded lines must have advance approval of appropriate dairy inspectors. Low-level pipeline systems, with the milk pipe at or below udder level, reduce excessive vacuum fluctuation at the claw or cup caused by vertical lift of the milk. Although it is difficult to install low lines in existing stanchion barns, all new barns and parlors should be designed for low-line systems. In general, milk-pipe systems in flat

barns should have no dead ends; that is, the milk pipe should be looped and both ends should enter the milk receiver through separate inlets. Normally, the high point in the loop would be at the most remote point from the receiver. In single-string barns, a simple loop should be installed. Larger barns require double (multiple) looped systems and/or larger milk pipes for optimum performance.

n) *Teat cups*. The teat cup consists of an outer shell, usually of stainless steel, and an inner liner or inflation. Liners are classed as molded, one-piece stretch, or ring-type stretch. Further specifications include wide (>19 mm inside diameter) or narrow bore and hardness or tensile characteristics (i.e., firm, medium, or soft). During the vacuum phase of the pulsation cycle, the liner opens and milk flows from the teat. Atmospheric air enters the outer chamber during the massage phase of the pulsation cycle, causing the liner to collapse against the teat end. The purpose of this action is to enhance circulation of blood through the tissues of the teat.

o) *Pulsator*. The pulsator is the automatic air-vacuum valve that directs atmospheric air into the chamber between the teat-cup liner and the shell and then withdraws this air by opening a port into the vacuum systems. This intermittent air-vacuum state causes the characteristic liner action. A master pulsator is designed to operate two or more milking units simultaneously, whereas a unit pulsator operates only one. Definite and somewhat snappy pulsator action is desirable. Unit pulsators near the teat cups give a sharp action by avoiding long pipes and hoses that can cause sluggish action caused by air friction. Slave, or booster, *unit* pulsators are used either to amplify or reproduce a weak, sluggish air-vacuum signal into a sharp action near the teat cups.

p) *Pulsation cycle*. Recorded measurements of vacuum in time and magnitude, made at the teat cup during milking with the system under full load, make possible the most comprehensive evaluation of milking machine performance. Teat-cup liners respond to the interaction of pulsated vacuum and milking vacuum. For this reason, critical determinations about milking depend on knowledge of both vacuums and an understanding of their interrelationships. Such measurements are recorded with the use of a strain gauge amplifier.

3. **Aquatic Animal Production**
   a) *Vertebrate fish production*
      1) *Total fish production worldwide*. In some areas of the world, including certain communities in the United States, fish are a significant part of the diet. If shellfish are included, fish production and harvesting on the global scale is actually greater than the combined production of beef, pork, and lamb. It is estimated that 700,000 *tons* a year are harvested from the sea for food, excluding large quantities of menhaden (used mainly for fish meal).
      2) *Commercial sources*. Two general types of vertebrate fish are processed commercially: saltwater and freshwater. Processing and distribution are essentially the same for both types. On the other hand, harvesting of the two has been entirely different. Saltwater fish are taken from the sea

with the aid of ships and their gear (capture fishing) or, more recently, by rearing fish such as salmon in enclosures. This practice, called *mariculture*, was originally associated only with oyster production. Today, *aquaculture* is used to describe farming of aquatic animals in either freshwater or saltwater. More than 8 million t of fish and shellfish are now produced by aquaculture.

3) *Saltwater fishing areas.* Currently, most saltwater capture fishing occurs in the northern hemisphere. Tropical oceans are not fished as heavily commercially because of preservation difficulties during transport. Even when a special effort is made to ensure adequate cooling, some deterioration occurs.

4) *Fish meal.* Fish may be processed for many uses. Most fish are sold directly as fresh, or fresh-frozen, table food. This industry has grown rapidly in recent years as a result of the development of new uses for the by-products of processing that utilize the fisherman's catch more completely. An excellent example is the use of fish in animal feeds. Menhaden, a fish commonly retrieved from the Atlantic Ocean, is the primary species used in fish meal production. Fish meal is an important source of protein and other nutrients for animal food supplements.

5) *Aquaculture worldwide.* Asia has approximately 80 percent of total aquaculture production worldwide, with China, Japan, Korea, and the Philippines the leading countries. Carp is the principal product. In Europe, France is the leading producer of rainbow trout and oysters. Norway is the leader in the rapidly expanding production of farm-raised Atlantic salmon, with significant industries also in Chile, Canada, Ireland, Iceland, and the Faroe Islands. Japan, Taiwan, Ecuador, and Brazil are current leaders in production of farmed-reared shrimp.

6) *Fish farms.* Two types of freshwater vertebrate fish currently farmed by aquaculture are catfish and trout. Channel catfish is the main vertebrate fish species farmed. This industry has grown remarkably in recent years. Rainbow trout is the principal trout species produced, with most production in Idaho and North Carolina. Salmon, and very recently striped bass, are saltwater species farmed. Salmon farming is located in Washington, Oregon, California, and Maine.

7) *Location of major catfish-processing plants.* Most United States catfish farming and processing is in the South and Midwest. In 1988, about 295 million lb of catfish were produced, representing a retail value of more than $270 million. Mississippi is currently the leading state with more than 62,000 acres in catfish ponds. Louisiana, Texas, Arkansas, Alabama, Tennessee, and Georgia are also major producers of catfish. Kansas, Florida, and California are involved to a lesser extent.

8) *Catfish farming.* Fish farming has become a complex operation. Initially ponds must be constructed and filled with water. Approved chemicals may be added to the water to control microbes. Temperature control of the water is especially critical when attempting to hatch eggs. A temperature of 26.6°C (80°F) appears to be best. Lower temperatures (21°C/70°F) retard hatching and enhance fungal growth on the eggs. Higher temperatures (32.2°C/90°F) permit eggs to hatch so rapidly that

they often deplete food supplies. Fish farms usually have separate ponds for hatching, raising fingerlings, and producing adult food fish.

9) *Major problems of the catfish farmer.* Ponds intended for harvesting catfish are stocked with fingerlings at the rate of about 2000/acre in the spring. Adult fish are harvested in the fall. The catfish farmer is constantly aware of two potential problems. Parasitic infestation of a pond can literally wipe out a crop of fish overnight; fortunately, some of these parasites can be controlled with approved chemicals. A second problem is that of oxygen depletion of the pond. When oxygen content becomes low (less than 3 ppm), oxygen must be added to the pond. This may be done by aeration or by adding fresh water.

10) *Harvesting and transporting catfish.* Catfish are harvested by combining two techniques, draining and seining. The fish, either alive or on ice, are then loaded on trucks and transported to the processing plant. Crushed ice is used to minimize bruising. A disadvantage of hauling live fish is that some may be injured in the loading process or die en route and contaminate the rest of the catch with postmortem body discharges. On the other hand, iced fish are more difficult to skin, their processing cannot be delayed, and icing is an added expense.

11) *Common methods used for harvesting saltwater fish.* Commercial saltwater fishing requires a general understanding of the habitat of the fish to be harvested. For example, some fish are found more frequently on the ocean bottom; catching them usually requires a net such as an otter trawl that is designed to pick up fish near the ocean floor. Other considerations regarding choice of gear include personal preference and, more important, the terrain of the ocean floor. If it is extremely rugged, line fishing may be necessary.

   (a) *Purse seine.* The purse seine, perhaps the most important piece of fishing gear used in the United States, is used commonly on both coasts to catch fish in the middle depths or close to the ocean surface. Important species caught include salmon, sardines, tuna, herring, and mackerel.

   (b) *Otter trawl and gill nets.* The otter trawl, the most common type of trawling gear, is used primarily for catching bottom-dwelling species such as cod, rockfish, and flatfish (e.g., flounder). A gill net is important in catching Pacific salmon. The size of the openings in the net varies depending on the type of fish to be harvested. The depth of the net is regulated by use of an anchor.

   (c) *Trolling.* In line fishing, the fisherman may troll or remain stationary. Commercial trolling is used most frequently by West Coast salmon and albacore fisheries. Stationary boats may use drift lines or set lines. Drift lines are popular with mackerel or tuna fishermen. Set lines are used primarily for catching halibut, black cod, rockfish, and other bottom dwellers.

b) *Shellfish production*

1) *Commercial shellfish sources.* Like vertebrate fish, some species of shellfish thrive in fresh water whereas others thrive in salt water. Shellfish of commercial importance are morphologically divided into two

general categories: mollusks (e.g., clams or oysters) and crustaceans (e.g., crawfish, shrimp or lobster).

2) *Crawfish*. Crawfish are the only freshwater shellfish of commercial importance. Other shellfish such as freshwater clams may be eaten occasionally but are not harvested commercially for food. Currently, about 500 species of crawfish exist throughout the world, with more than 250 occurring in North America.

3) *Crawfish farming in the United States*. Commercial production of crawfish involves aquaculture similar to raising catfish. In the United States most crawfish farming is in Louisiana. In 1987, the annual United States crawfish harvest was estimated at 95 million lb, with a value of more than $70 million. Crawfish farming had an accidental beginning about 1950, when a farmer flooded a rice field in the fall to develop a temporary area for duck hunting. The next spring the pond was teeming with crawfish. Subsequently, the idea of crawfish farming evolved. This concept has been applied since to catfish and some saltwater shellfish. Coastal water shrimp farming (mariculture) is an example of applying fish farming to seafood production. In years to come, aquaculture will probably become extremely important in supplying the nutritional needs of the United States.

4) *Types of crawfish ponds*. Two types of ponds are used in farming crawfish. Rice fields are popular in rice-growing areas. The general procedure involves draining the rice field 2 wk before rice harvest. As the fields dry, crawfish burrow into the soil. Later, a second growth of rice, grasses, etc., provides food for the developing crawfish. Wooded areas also are used to make ponds. This latter type of pond is less desirable as it tends to become low in oxygen because wind-aided water circulation is poor. Also, wooded areas are usually more acid, which is not conducive to crawfish production. Nevertheless, these ponds are popular because they allow use of land that otherwise would be idle.

5) *Crawfish farming procedures*. Crawfish farming simply involves stocking the pond with brood stock. The number of crawfish stocked depends on the amount of vegetation available. Stocking usually is done in May or June. About a month later, the ponds are drained to induce burrowing of the crawfish. The ponds are flooded in the fall, which results in the release of young crawfish. The young adult crawfish then feed on vegetation until they are harvested. Depending on climatic conditions, adults may be harvested from late November through April.

6) *Crawfish harvesting*. Crawfish currently are harvested by hand with the use of lift nets or funnel traps. The live crawfish are kept in holding tanks and transported to processing plants where they are stored in coolers at 3.3°C (38°F).

7) *Oysters*. Oysters are the primary commercially marketed mollusks in the United States. Most oysters harvested in this country are from the Atlantic Ocean and the Gulf of Mexico. Although oysters are present in the Pacific, overharvesting in the past has made the West Coast a less-important source today.

8) *Oyster beds*. Oysters prefer a habitat of brackish water at depths down

to 40–50 ft (12–15 m). Although they grow in deeper waters, there are no important oyster beds harvested commercially at depths greater than 40 ft (12 m). Oysters require a fairly hard surface on which to thrive but are little affected by fluctuations in water temperature and salinity. Because the floor of the Gulf of Mexico tends to become muddy from river drainage, shells from processed oysters are used to provide a hard surface on which to grow newly seeded oysters.

9) *Commercial production of oysters.* Oysters are harvested commercially from either of two sites: (1) public grounds regulated by strict conservation rules that control methods of harvesting, amounts harvested, etc., and (2) private grounds managed by individuals who reseed the bed after harvesting.

10) *Mollusk harvesting.* Mollusks may be harvested by several methods, depending on the species and the harvester's preference. Often, only hand-harvesting methods are allowed in public waters because mechanical dredgers tend to overharvest. Since most oysters in the United States are farmed in private waters, dredges are popular. Dredged oysters tend to be cleaner than tonged oysters because they are washed as they are brought out of the water and onto the boat.

11) *Clams.* Several species of clam are harvested commercially. Procedures used to harvest and process clams are essentially the same as those for oysters. More hand-harvesting of clams is done than of oysters because some species inhabit shallow waters. Hard-shell and ocean quahog clams prefer shallow oceanic shores, thus requiring the use of tongs. On the other hand, soft-shell clams are found primarily in estuarine waters. Hand-harvesting with a pail and shovel when the tide is out is the principal method used with important commercial species. Because of their larger size, there is more meat yield. These clams inhabit the deeper waters of the North Atlantic states, thus requiring dredging rigs for harvesting. Harvested clams remain alive for fairly long periods by closing their shells tightly to conserve moisture. Large clams, such as the surf clam, are marketed as a canned product either whole or minced; smaller sizes are usually sold fresh for steaming or on the half shell.

12) *Sea and bay scallops.* Scallops are another commercially important mollusk. Two types of scallops are harvested: sea and bay scallop. Sea scallops reside in deep ocean water and must be retrieved by dredging or with the otter trawl. Bay scallops may be harvested by hand since they are in shallow waters. Scallops must be handled carefully when harvested because, unlike other mollusks, they cannot close their shells tightly after removal from the water and consequently dry out and die quickly. Most sea scallops are shucked on board ship. Scallop processing and marketing is essentially the same as for other mollusks.

13) *Commercially marketed saltwater crustaceans.* Shrimp, crab, and lobster are the principal commercial species of saltwater crustaceans. Shrimp are harvested from most U.S. coastal waters. The large shrimp, which are the most important commercially, come from the Gulf of Mexico.

14) *Commercial crab harvesting.* Three important species of crabs are harvested in U.S. coastal waters: the Dungeness and king crabs of the

Pacific and the blue crab of the Atlantic. Several types of gear are used to harvest crabs. *Trot lines* (baited lines with no hook) are used primarily for hard crabs. Wading fishermen may pass push nets or dip nets on poles in shallow waters. Crab pots, popular for harvesting blue and Dungeness crabs, are simply baited traps placed on the ocean floor.

15) *Lobsters*. Lobsters harvested from U.S. coastal waters are taken primarily from the north and, to some extent, the middle Atlantic. Their habitat is on the ocean bottom from the shoreline to the edge of the continental shelf. Although lobsters do not migrate great distances, they will move to and from shore in search of food.

Lobster pots are used to catch lobsters, which are drawn to the baited trap in search of food. Most lobsters are marketed alive. Lobsters can live up to 7 mo without food. Lobsters (whole or tails) usually are frozen raw rather than cooked, as lobsters frozen after cooking tend to be less tender.

16) *Controlled shellfishing areas*. Shellfish can be a threat to public health because many communities dump sewage in coastal waters, which are often (along with adjacent areas) the habitat for shellfish. It is essential, therefore, that sewage treatment plants effectively destroy or remove any pathogenic agents that can pass through the food chain. In reality, this is a very difficult task. The Shellfish Sanitation Branch of the Division of Environmental Engineering and Food Protection (USPHS) provides a partial solution to this problem by its control of harvesting areas.

B. PROCESSING

Objectives

1. Plant Construction, Equipment, and Sanitation
    a) Describe three basic requirements of materials used in constructing or equipping a sanitary facility.
    b) Explain design features and efficacy of various materials used in the construction of floors, ceilings, walls, and equipment that involve sanitation.
    c) Outline steps in a water potability test and interpret results.
    d) Identify resources for practitioners who need or wish to have water samples examined for chemical constituents.
    e) Describe the two basic elements of a satisfactory pest-control program.
    f) Describe how to evaluate the effectiveness of a pest-control program.
    g) Describe sanitary dressing procedures and methods to preclude contamination of food materials in red meat plants.

2. Meat Processing and Preservation
    a) Describe meat-processing procedures and identify activities that are potential sources of contamination.
    b) Explain the procedures used in preserving wholesomeness of meat and meat products.

3. Control of Inedible and Condemned Products

a) Describe inedible and condemned materials and the health hazards associated with the consumption of these materials.
b) Describe methods to dispose of these materials properly.
c) Describe the environmental health hazards associated with improper disposal of these materials.
d) Describe how these materials may be misused.

4. Poultry Processing
   a) Describe the essentials of modern poultry processing.
   b) Describe procedures and potential for contamination in relation to transportation, slaughtering, defeathering, and processing.

5. Pasteurization of Milk
   a) Define milk pasteurization.
   b) State two objectives (purposes) of pasteurization.
   c) Explain the rationale for the time-temperature relationships for LTH, HTST, and UHT pasteurization.
   d) Explain equipment features of the LTH, HTST, and UHT methods that ensure effectiveness of pasteurization.
   e) Explain the salt conductivity test and alkaline phosphatase analysis in evaluating pasteurization effectiveness.
   f) Explain the significance of coliform bacteria in pasteurized milk.
   g) Describe potential health hazards associated with manufactured dairy products.

6. Aquatic Animal Processing
   a) Describe the essentials of modern fishing processing.
   b) Describe the essentials of modern processing of edible crustaceans and mollusks.

Text

1. Plant Construction, Equipment, and Sanitation
   a) Three basic characteristics are necessary for building material or equipment in a food-handling facility. They must be *impervious* to chemicals and microorganisms, *resistant to wear and corrosion,* and *easy to clean*. Standards for meat-processing-plant construction and equipment are established by the United States Department of Agriculture (USDA).
   1) *Floors.* The floor is perhaps the most significant item to consider in constructing a facility in which sanitation is important. All matter falls to the floor, and unless a floor is properly constructed and maintained, it can create a serious problem. No other surface is exposed to such intense wear, so durability is a prime factor. In addition, floors are cleaned and disinfected so the construction must be free from depressions, cracks, and separations.

   Concrete is an excellent flooring material when properly installed. It may crack, however, allowing food scraps and microorganisms to collect even with routine cleaning. The texture of the concrete is also important. Fat, grease, or even water can make a smooth floor slippery and a hazard to employees. A floor that is too coarse is difficult to clean adequately.

Brick also makes good flooring when properly installed. The brick must be of good quality, and it must be laid over a concrete base and bonded with an acid-resistant and waterproof mortar.

Wood floors, although occasionally found in processing rooms and coolers of some older plants, are not preferred. Wood is unacceptable where water is used. If the wood floor is free from cracks and can be kept clean, it may be used in selected areas. Nevertheless, wood is one of the least satisfactory materials for flooring.

Synthetic poured floors are especially good because they have no seams. They can even be installed to include walls and ceiling as well as the floor, thus forming a completely seamless room. The materials used most commonly are epoxy or fiberglass plastics; both are quite expensive. They may be used to upgrade an unacceptable wood floor since they can be installed over the old floor, which is more economical than removing the old floor and installing a base of another type. However, adequate preparation of the old surface is very important.

2) *Walls.* A smooth, flat, impervious material is most satisfactory for interior wall construction. Materials such as brick, tile, or plaster are satisfactory. Unacceptable wall materials absorb moisture or are hard to clean, such as wood, plasterboard, or porous acoustical board. Concrete block is less desirable because it is difficult to clean, although it is commonly used. Latex or rubberized paints applied to the block wall make it acceptable.

Coving (curved base plate) at the junction between the wall and floor is a desirable construction feature for any health facility. Sanitation of coved rooms is decidedly easier.

Bumper guards prevent damage to the wall by carts, trucks, etc. Chipped or damaged walls are difficult to clean. Esthetically appealing guards can be used in areas where public traffic is heavy.

3) *Ceilings.* Although ceilings are not usually exposed to direct physical wear and corrosion, they may serve as a source of contamination. Consequently, they should be constructed of a material that does not chip, peel, deteriorate, or retain dust or condensation.

4) *Equipment.* Equipment design and materials are important to minimize contamination. Rounded corners and lack of seams help eliminate places for growth of microorganisms. Stainless steel is used to handle food products because it is cleaned easily and is resistant to wear and corrosion.

Plastics of an approved type may be used in several places in processing plants. Ease of cleaning is a primary criterion. Galvanized metal may be used in certain areas of the plant. It is not as resistant to corrosion as stainless steel, however, so it must be used judiciously.

Cutting boards are necessary in meat-processing plants. A board may be constructed of single-piece hardwood or of an approved plastic or rubber-plastic combination. Laminated cutting boards or chopping blocks are unacceptable because the laminations tend to separate, especially when hot water is used in cleaning, permitting juices and small pieces of meat to lodge in the openings and become sources of contamination.

The small-tool sanitizer is required in slaughtering plants to minimize cross-contamination with infectious agents. The sanitizer maintains water at a temperature of 82.2°C (180°F). After use on animals or anytime there is obvious contamination, the knives, hooks, and saws are dipped into the sanitizer. The sanitizer temperature exceeds the thermal death point of 76.7°C (170°F) for most mesophilic organisms. Most pathogenic bacteria are mesophilic. If a knife or other equipment to be sanitized is contaminated grossly with purulent exudate, dirt, or hair, it should be washed in water before sanitizing.

5) *Water potability*

   (a) *Periodic analysis.* All sources of water used on or around food in a slaughter plant must be examined periodically for contamination by pathogenic microorganisms or toxic chemicals to ensure compliance with established standards. City water as well as water from each well used by the plant must be included in this evaluation. If nonpotable water is used in areas where there is no danger of contamination of food, the pipes carrying this water must be identified clearly to avoid cross-connections with the potable supply. Samples of water from each source are obtained at representative points throughout the system. When sampling from a tap, the water should be allowed to run freely for 2-3 min to allow sufficient time to clear the line. Less than 2.2 coliforms/100 ml, based on five 10-ml samples, is generally considered acceptable.

   (b) *Detailed analysis.* When a veterinary practitioner must obtain a more detailed analysis of a water source, several facilities are available. A state animal diagnostic laboratory or some unit in a state university usually will be able to analyze water samples for normal mineral constituents as well as the presence of potentially hazardous chemicals. These types of laboratories normally provide this service without charge but restrict their work to investigations involving food animals.

   For a fee, most private laboratories will perform work for practitioners, regardless of the species of animal involved.

6) *Pest control*

   (a) *Elements.* It is impossible to permanently eliminate all pests in facilities that prepare or store food. Control is the best that can be achieved and depends on two elements: environmental sanitation and effective chemical and physical control.

   Environmental sanitation involves proper refuse and garbage storage and removal, employee education programs, and daily sanitation inspections.

   Effective physical and chemical control involves the use of barriers, such as screening, to prevent entry of pests into the establishment, as well as the proper use of chemicals and physical traps to control pests that have gained entry. This requires efficient utilization of approved pesticides and a familiarity with the life cycle and behavior patterns of the various species. As in environmental sanitation, frequent inspection is necessary to maintain effective control. Chemicals used in pest- and rodent-control programs in food-processing facilities must be restricted to those compounds approved for such use.

(b) *Effectiveness*. The results of a pest-control program are evaluated by searching for physical evidence of infestation. For most insect species, this is achieved by noting their presence in the food-handling establishment. Flies are usually obvious and cockroaches less so, and beetles and moths usually require an examination of the food to detect their presence. Rodents usually are detected by recognition of various signs that can indicate not only the species but the severity of the infestation. Some of these signs follow:

Droppings are one of the best indications of infestation. Rat droppings are large, up to 2 cm (3/4 in.), with blunt ends.

Burrows can be rat holes approximately 7.5 cm (3 in.), in diameter or mouse holes about 2.5 cm (1 in.) in diameter. An active burrow is free of cobwebs and dust.

Tracks, which are more clearly discerned by side illumination from a flashlight, may be observed anywhere along rat or mouse runs. Dust and soft mud are especially good places to observe tracks.

Grease streaks on walls indicate runs.

7) *Sanitary dressing procedures*

(a) *Cattle*. In modern large-volume slaughtering plants, carcasses are shackled by the hind legs and attached to a moving overhead chain powered by electric motors. In some smaller-volume plants, the dressing procedure starts on the floor with the carcass positioned on its back by pritch poles. Regardless of the method used, great care must be take to prevent contamination during dressing.

The first step is removal of the hide. This is usually accomplished with pneumatic knives and in most large establishments with some type of mechanical hide-puller. Fecal material on the skin may be a source of carcass contamination, and washing cattle before slaughter will not reduce this problem.

After the head is skinned and removed, the hooves are removed and the animal is skinned. The head is cleaned with a high-pressure hose, marked with a tag bearing the same number as the carcass, and set aside for inspection.

After the skin, head, and feet have been removed, the carcass is positioned next to a long, metal moving table and eviscerated. The viscera are placed adjacent to the carcass so that the inspector can relate one to the other. This is the second point in the dressing procedure with very high potential for contamination. During evisceration, great care must be exercised to prevent soiling the carcass with material from the gastrointestinal tract. The rectum is dissected free and tied off with a piece of string (a procedure called "dropping the bung") before the abdominal cavity is opened. Seepage of material from the anterior end of the gastrointestinal tract is prevented by separating the esophagus from the trachea and tying it off (a process referred to as "rodding the weasand"). The moving table surface (which is also chain-driven) is automatically steam-cleaned before reuse.

After the viscera and carcass have been inspected and passed, the edible portions of the viscera are separated from the inedible and the carcass split into two halves along the spinal column, washed and covered with a muslin sheet (called "shrouding"), and chilled in a cooler until ready to be cut up.

(b) *Sheep and goats*. Dressing procedures for these species are similar to those for cattle except that skinning is done entirely by hand and requires more care to prevent contamination.

(c) *Swine*. The first step following slaughter is immersion in a scald vat to facilitate hair removal. Two things may occur at this point that will result in carcass condemnation: (1) If a pig is not completely bled out, asphyxiation occurs, and (2) some carcasses may drop off the moving chain and become cooked in the scald vat, making the skin so friable that it will tear, which results in gross contamination of underlying tissues.

After the carcasses leave the scald vat, they pass through a dehairing machine that consists of a large, metal, revolving cylinder lined with rubber-surfaced paddles. These paddles, moving at high speed, rub the hair off the softened skin. The roughness of this procedure may express fecal material from some carcasses, resulting in contamination. Use of chlorinated wash water to flush the hair and debris from these machines during use helps to alleviate this problem.

After dehairing, the dressing procedure is similar to that of ruminants except that finished carcasses are not shrouded before being placed in the cooler.

2. Meat Processing and Preservation
a) *Processing procedure*
1) *Offal*. In red meat plants, the term *offal* refers to edible parts of the animal *other than* the carcass. Sometimes, when loosely applied, edible offal used solely in reference to edible viscera. In poultry plants, offal refers to inedible parts of the bird.

When offal is retrieved from the animal, there is considerable opportunity for contamination. For example, as it is removed from the body, offal may contact the animal's hide. Furthermore, since the intestinal tract is inherently contaminated, it is not surprising that microorganisms exist in high numbers in the environment of this area of the plant.

The offal-processing area is an excellent environment for the spread of contaminating microorganisms. Water freely used in offal processing further distributes microorganisms. Since the animals were killed only minutes before, the temperature of the offal is conducive to microbial multiplication. Also, animal tissue is an excellent source of nutrients for growth of microorganisms.

It is especially important to process offal products without delay. Rapid processing ensures minimal microbial multiplication.

Processing of some of the more commonly used edible offal is reviewed below. For description of other offal products, refer to meat hygiene texts.

(a) *Liver*. This is one of the more commonly processed offal products. Normal processing involves removal of the gall bladder, hepatic and portal lymph nodes, and excess fat. Normally, the liver has been inspected before it reaches the offal area.

(b) *Beef hearts*. These also are saved as edible offal. Initial inspection is done during postmortem examination on the kill floor. At that time, the ventricles are incised and inspected. It is not until offal inspection, however, that the organ is examined by palpation as well as visually.

(c) *Pork hearts*. Pork hearts are handled somewhat differently. The organ is examined only externally at postmortem. It is not until offal inspection that the heart is incised and inspected internally. Before offal inspection, pork hearts are sent through a slasher. In dealing with either beef or pork hearts, it is essential to remove clotted blood. Failure to do so shortens shelf life remarkably.

(d) *Beef and pork tongues*. These are saved for food by many processors. Before offal inspection, tonsillar tissue should be inspected and removed. Once the tongue and oropharyngeal tissues have been removed from the head, the tonsils are difficult to identify. Inspection of the tongue includes visual observation for ulcers and lacerations. Palpation is important to detect abnormalities. Tongue worms and abscesses are important considerations when examining pork tongues. After tongues of either species are examined, they are scalded.

(e) *Head muscle*. This is valuable to the large processor because many products can be made from this tissue. In cattle, muscle from the cheek and poll areas often is salvaged. Offal inspection allows a second opportunity to examine for lesions indicating conditions commonly associated with this tissue (e.g., cysticercosis, eosinophilic myositis).

(f) *Beef tails*. Beef tails (commonly called ox tails) are saved routinely by most plants. Contamination during hair removal is a major problem. Bruising is usually a sequela of vertebral fractures. Consequently, much trimming may be necessary before this product can be marketed.

(g) *Kidneys*. These usually are saved for food. If a lesion is noted, however, the entire organ is discarded.

(h) *Blood*. In certain areas of the country, blood sausage is a much-desired product. Sanitary collection is imperative if blood is to be salvaged. Collection involves the use of anticoagulants and a defibrinating machine. Citrate is a commonly used anticongulant. Sanitary collection is more important than the amount of citrate used since this anticoagulant is essentially nontoxic to the consumer. Blood is an excellent medium for bacteria, so it is an important potential health hazard. Hog blood cannot be used.

(i) *Tripe.* This is another tissue classed as edible offal. It includes the rumen and reticulum. The first step in processing this product is to open the rumen and discard its contents. After the contents have been removed, the rumen and reticulum are hung in an umbrella fashion over a large conical structure. Subsequently, contaminated areas on the serosal surface are trimmed and the remainder washed. Following washing, tripe is placed in a large tumbler machine. The tumbling and turning, in conjunction with scalding, help to remove the mucosa. After the mucosa is removed, the tripe is bleached and rinsed. Scalding, tumbling, bleaching, and rinsing all take place in the same tumbler. Finally, the product may be cooked. The term *honeycomb* refers to the appearance of the reticulum.

(j) *Chitterlings.* Swine large intestine (chitterlings) is another tissue classed as edible offal. Processing involves removal of fecal contents (stripping), splitting, washing, cleaning, and chilling. It is virtually impossible to remove all fecal contamination from these products.

(k) *Beef and pork brains.* These may be saved for food, depending on the stunning procedure employed. Sometime, even with an efficacious method, subdural hemorrhage occurs and the brain must be condemned.

(l) *Pork stomachs.* When used for food, pork stomachs are processed similarly to other intestinal viscera. The contents are first removed and then the stomach is washed. Later it is heated in a vat at about 48.9°C (120°F). This enables easy removal of the mucosa, which before heating has the appearance of slime. Next it is rinsed and scalded. Finally, after inspection, the stomach is chilled.

2) *Sausage production.* Sausage is a comminuted product composed of meat or meat food products that are seasoned with condimental substances, excluding eggs, vegetables, gelatins, macaronis, cheese, and pickles, and which may contain certain additives in permitted amounts. The product may be marketed fresh, cooked, cooked and smoked, semidry, or dry. Several compounds are added to sausage as preservatives, curing agents, flavor enhancers, color fixatives, or expanders. Their use must be controlled to ensure that the final product does not contain excessive amounts.

In the United States, 85 percent of the sausage is marketed in the cooked or smoked form; of this, about 55 percent of retail sales are frankfurters or wieners. Sausage production may vary with the type of sausage produced and the size of the operation.

(a) *Batching.* This is the initial step in sausage production. All of the ingredients to be incorporated into the sausage are set out in the correct proportions before actual processing.

(b) *Grinding*. Next the meat is ground to the desired texture (course or fine).

(c) *Mixing*. This step can be done by hand, or with the aid of a mechanical mixer. All the ingredients included in the final product are mixed at this time.

(d) *Binding power*. The binding power of the mixture must be considered so that the final emulsion does not fall apart. The primary consideration is containing the fatty portion of the mixture. Fat globules are bound by myosin, a protein that is effective in holding the mixture together. Myosin will lose its ability to tie up fat globules if the mixture is overheated. Generally, binding power is lost at temperatures above 21.1°C (70°F). This is why ice often is added to the mixture before curing.

(e) *Curing*. After the ingredients have been mixed, the product is placed in a container to cure.

(f) *Stuffing*. After the product is cured, it is ready for stuffing into the casing. Usually casings are filled with the emulsion under pressure and tied at regular lengths. Today many casings are made of synthetics such as cellulose. Although less common today, natural casings (intestines) are used to give a sausage a homemade appearance.

(g) *Cooking or smoking*. The product is now ready for cooking or smoking. Most often, smoking is preferred because of the flavor imparted. The procedure is normally performed in large, walk-in ovens with precise time and temperature controls.

(h) *Showering*. In the final step in sausage production, water is sprayed on the product to cool it and prevent bacterial growth. This rapid cooling process also prevents excessive water loss from the product and therefore helps to minimize shrinkage.

b) *Preservation procedures*. Concern for meat preservation is primarily related to two phenomena: microbial contamination and autolytic changes at the cellular level. Five general methods can be used to preserve a product and increase its shelf life: heat, cold, dehydration, irradiation, or addition of chemicals. Any of these techniques effectively minimize the deleterious changes caused by microorganisms or autolysis.

1) *Heat*. Heat is the method used most commonly to preserve food. In applying heat, such as in cooking meat before canning, one must be aware that products and microorganisms both vary in their heat susceptibility. Consequently the optimal temperature for preserving meat products must be established to eliminate putrefactive and pathogenic microorganisms, most of which are destroyed at temperatures greater than 60°C (140°F). Heat can be applied to a product in several ways. Moist heat in the form of boiling water or steam generally is more effective than dry heat because moist heat is more penetrating. Fatty foods are an exception.

(a) *Canning*. Canning utilizes heat to render a product *commercially sterile*. This means that the consumer can store the product for an indefinite period without taking special precautions. The canning process uses destruction of nontoxic putrefactive clostridia as the standard to measure effectiveness of the process; the highly toxigenic anaerobic microorganism *Clostridium botulinum* is less resistant to heat than the more saprophytic members of the genus, so killing the latter ensures that all botulinum-toxin-producing organisms are killed. The thermal death time of the organisms varies, depending on the temperature and pressure utilized. Therefore, it is imperative that the conditions of temperature, pressure, and time be established to ensure that the canning procedure is effective.

Some products, such as canned ham, cannot be heated to temperatures that render them sterile because of a loss in quality from overcooking. Pasteurized or partially sterilized products are heated to a temperature of approximately 71.1°C (160°F) to kill surface organisms. Because these products are not sterile, they must be kept refrigerated. Prepackaged luncheon meat is another example of a pasteurized meat product. Curing agents, which inhibit bacterial growth, can be used to advantage in preparing cooked food products. Curing products are incorporated into the meat products, allowing them to be cooked at a lower temperature. The benefit of using curing agents is that products such as ham, sensitive to higher temperatures, have an improved shelf life.

(b) *Smoking.* Some foods because of their inherent lower pH, can be processed and canned at lower temperatures. Spores in acids are less resistant to heat and can be destroyed at lower temperatures. Smoking, a procedure in which the meat product is exposed to the smoke generated by the slow burning of various hardwoods, most popularly hickory, is another method to preserve a meat product.

Smoking is effective in preserving meat for two reasons: (1) it dries the meat surface and thus inhibits oxidation, and (2) smoke deposits phenolic compounds on the surface that inhibit fat oxidation. Many processors, however, add water during the smoking process in amounts that reduce drying and thus the bacteriostatic effect. In commercial processing the internal temperature of the meat product is usually brought high enough to kill potential pathogens without any assistance from the smoke.

2) *Cold*

(a) *Cold storage.* Cold is a second means of preserving meat. Once a meat-product temperature has been lowered to 4.4°C (40°F), most pathogens do not grow. However, most microorganisms are not killed by the lower temperature. When a carcass is put into a cooler, not only is the meat preserved, but potential pathogens are preserved also! This is a weak link in the processing chain.

While the carcass is being cooled to its storage temperature, humidity must be maintained in the range of 88–92 percent because slime mold is more likely to form on its surface at relative humidities greater than 92 percent and shrinkage will occur at less than 88 percent.

Cold storage in the range of 0°–1.7°C (32°–35°F) is most effective in preserving meat products. Experiments at various temperatures have demonstrated that frankfurters, for instance, last up to 4 times longer when kept at 0°C (32°F) compared with 10°C (50°F). During the cutting and wrapping process, meat should be kept at 0°C (32°F). Complete freezing during processing is not desirable because repeated freezing and thawing has a deleterious effect on meat flavor.

Curing uncooked meats is an excellent aid to preservation by refrigeration. Curing salts inhibit psychrophilic organisms, so the resulting product is more stable. Normally curing salts alone will not inhibit all contaminating microorganisms. Thus cured products should be refrigerated. It is unnecessary to freeze cured meats since they last for a relatively long time under refrigeration. Actually, freezing cured meats tends to increase the likelihood of rancid fat.

(b) *Freezing*. This is an excellent method of preserving foods. The rate at which meat is frozen influences its quality. If the freezing process occurs slowly, larger ice crystals form between muscle fibers and the resulting product is of poorer quality because of cell membrane damage and concomitant leakage of intracellular elements. Consequently, meat should be frozen rapidly. Usually meat is frozen to −23.3°C (−10°F) and then stored at −17°C (0.0°F).

Pork products cannot be maintained frozen as long as beef because of the relatively higher amounts of unsaturated fats in pork. With time, the unsaturated fats are oxidized.

3) *Dehydration*. Dehydration, a third general method of meat preservation, is effective for two reasons: (1) enzymatic processes within cells are slowed, thereby retarding autolytic changes, and (2) lack of moisture in the meat is unfavorable for bacterial growth. Dehydration can be accomplished by either hot-air-drying or freeze-drying.

(a) *Hot-air-drying*. This is an old method, used by American Indians to produce beef jerky. Residual moisture content of hot-air-dried meat is about 5.0 percent whereas moisture in freeze-dried meat is reduced to 1.0 percent.

Hot-air-drying preserves meats up to 12 mo before signs of deterioration appear. A disadvantage of this method is that fatty meats such as pork tend to become rancid unless an antioxidant is added during cooking and the product is well wrapped after final processing to prevent exposure to air. Another disadvantage is that raw meat cannot be dehydrated by this means.

(b) *Freeze-drying*. Freeze-drying, on the other hand, effectively preserves both cooked and raw meat. Shelf life varies depending on the ambient temperature. Special precautions are needed with meats high in fat.

4) *Irradiation*. This is the fourth method of preservation. As ionizing radiation is passed through a living cell, electrons are ejected, changing the atomic structure and causing cell death.

(a) *Definitions*

(1) *Kilogray.* One kilogray (kGy) equals 100 kilorads (krad). (One rad equals 100 ergs of energy absorbed per gram of absorber.)

(2) *Disinfestation.* This is treatment at doses to destroy insects.

(3) *Radappertization.* This is treatment at sterilizing doses to destroy all organisms.

(4) *Radicidation.* This is treatment at pasteurizing doses to inactivate non-spore-forming pathogens.

(5) *Radurization.* This is treatment at doses to destroy spoilage organisms.

(b) *History.* As early as 1921, a U.S. patent was issued for using X rays to destroy trichinae in pork. By 1947, advances in equipment design had made it possible to preserve a variety of foods but commercial applications were limited because of poor penetration of tissue. In 1963, the U.S. Army established a laboratory at Natick, Massachusetts, which was equipped with a cobalt-60 irradiator and a high-energy electron generator. Since then, similar facilities have been established throughout the world.

(c) *Legislation.* In the United States, radiation is considered to be an "additive" to food rather than a process and is subject to federal regulations under the Food, Drug, and Cosmetic Act, Title 21, Part 179. Section 201 (s) defines an additive as "any substance the intended use of which, results . . . in its becoming a component or otherwise affecting the characteristic of any food . . . and including any source of radiation intended for any such use."

(d) *Procedures.* Radiation may be applied as X rays, as electron bombardment, or as gamma rays. X rays can be generated from sources not to exceed 5 million electron volts, electrons from generators not to exceed 10 million volts, and gamma rays from sealed units of the isotopes cobalt-60 or cesium-137.

The primary advantage of X rays and electron beams over isotopes is that, being machine generated, they can easily be switched on and off as the need arises. Isotope irradiators emit and decay constantly and, unless heavily used, have reduced economic return. The disadvantages of X-ray and electron beam generators are high cost and low penetrating power. Effective irradiation is limited to small, low-density items (under 0.2 g/cm^3) and sliced meat or fish up to 5 cm thick.

Cobalt-60, with a half-life of 5.3 yr, is more commonly used in multipurpose irradiation units than cesium-137, which has a half-life of 30 yr, because the source strength of the latter has to be considerably higher to achieve equal results. In small, low-dose, mobile irradiators, where weight is an important consideration, cesium-137 is favored because of the lower amount of shielding required.

See Table 1.2 for current applications.

5) *Chemicals.* Adding chemicals, called *curing agents,* is the fifth general method for preservation of meat products. Some caution must be exercised in the choice of chemicals. For example, many bactericidal

Table 1.2. Current applications of irradiation in food preservation

Effect	Product	Dose
Sprout inhibition	Potatoes, onions, garlic	10 to 20 kGy
Modifying ripening and improving quality	Papayas, avocados, tropical fruit	0.1 to 1 kGy
Disinfestation	Grains, cereals, fruits, spices	0.3 to 1 kGy
Radurization to extend shelf-life of products	Meat, seafood, vegetables, fruit	0.5 to 10 kGy
Radicidation to eliminate bacterial pathogens	Meat, fish, seafood	1 to 10 kGy
Radappertization to achieve sterilization	Meat, fish, seafood, spices	10 to 50 kGy

compounds are so toxic that they cannot be used as food preservatives.

(a) *Water*. Although *water* is not a curing agent, it is the largest single ingredient of any curing preparation. Since the curing preparation often is injected into the product, only potable water should be utilized. Water may increase the yield of the final product, but it does not enhance the flavor, tenderness, etc.

(b) *Salt*. Sodium chloride is an effective bacteriostatic agent. Inhibition of microbial growth is achieved by the increased osmotic pressure of salt in the medium, although there is considerable variability among microorganisms in sensitivity to salt. Salt is also used for its flavor-enhancing effect.

(c) *Nitrite and nitrate salts*. These salts have been used in curing as color fixatives as well as preservatives. The two salts often have been used concurrently. Nitrite aids in providing a rapid initial cure whereas nitrate provides a source of nitrite during storage. Nitrates must be converted to nitrites to be effective. These agents are highly toxic if ingested in excessive quantities. Since under certain conditions nitrates break down into potentially carcinogenic nitrosamines, use of nitrates in curing mixes is no longer permitted.

(d) *Sugar*. The main purpose of adding sugar is to help reduce the harsh flavor that salt adds to a product. Sugars are useful in providing a favorable medium for growth of desirable flavor-producing bacteria. Product yield is increased somewhat by added sugar.

(e) *Phosphates*. These are included as an adjunct to curing agents to improve the water-holding capability of the product. Although the mechanism has not been established, intracellular proteins are known to increase water-binding capacity with a concomitant increase in pH. Addition of phosphates is self-limiting since, in excess, they precipitate out of the brine solution and crystallize on the meat. In excess they can be toxic, so their use is restricted.

(f) *Ascorbates*. These are used as adjuncts to curing agents. These compounds effectively aid in fixing the color of products and thus prevent fading. Ascorbates have only minimal bacteriostatic effect on spoilage and mold-producing organisms. Therefore, amounts necessary for effective microbial control are excessive and would constitute adulteration.

(g) *Acids*. Certain acids may be used as bacteriostatic agents. Lactic and acetic acid are used commonly for this purpose as well as for flavor enhancement. Lactic acid bacilli are used routinely as starter cultures in certain foods or are added directly. It is this acid that gives such foods a tangy taste. As the pH of the acid decreases, a dramatic increase in bacteriostasis occurs. A decrease of 1 pH unit increases the bacteriostasis 10-fold.

(h) *Gases*. Carbon dioxide and ozone are effective meat preservatives. Carbon dioxide sometimes is used in the holds of large ships that are transporting whole carcasses. The gas acts to retard surface contaminant growth.

Ozone is emitted from ozone lamps. The gas has a bactericidal action on airborne microorganisms. This preservation technique has had limited use and must be used with discretion because of several disadvantages. (1) Ozone has an odor that masks any abnormal odors associated with meat aging. Consequently, substantial financial loss is possible. (2) At excessively high concentrations, ozone is hazardous to human health. (3) The gas also tends to accelerate development of fat rancidity.

(i) *Control of curing ingredients*. There are no legal limits on amounts of sodium chloride or sugars that can be used in curing. These compounds are self-limiting because of taste. There is some variability in the use of sugars. For example, maltose and lactose have low sweetening ability, so they can be added in greater quantities before the product becomes too sweet. Therefore, these compounds often are used as fillers.

(j) *Applying curing agents*. External application involves applying either a dry or liquid form of an agent. Although this method is still used, it has been generally discarded because of poor penetration. Curing agents are more effective if they are injected into a major vessel or into the tissue (called "stitch pumping"). Modern plants have multi-needled pumpers. Processors have sought more efficient methods of curing meat products than external application. Although greater penetration is achieved by injection, the processor still is required to retain the product while it cures. Several alternative methods have been attempted. One such method allows the curing reaction to occur within a sealed package. For example, individual bacon slices are passed through a warm (10°–15°C/50°–77°F) curing solution, drained, heated, and then packaged. The product is packaged in a hermetically sealed container and allowed to cure while on its way to the retailer.

(k) *Trichina control.* Since many cured products are from swine and often are processed as ready-to-eat, a potential health hazard exists because encysted trichina larvae are transmitted readily in products that are not prepared properly. Trichina cysts are killed when an internal temperature of 58.3°C (137°F) is achieved. Pork may be certified as trichina-free if it is frozen at −40°C (−40°F). Cysts of *Trichinella spiralis* are killed instantly at this temperature. For products such as dried sausage, salting and drying will destroy trichinae, but the time required varies with the amount of salt used and how fast the drying procedure is accomplished.

3. **Control of Inedible and Condemned Products**
    a) *Inedible products*
        1) *Categories. Inedible* materials are those that are not normally used for human food (bones, lungs, etc.). *Condemned* materials are those that would normally have been used for food but have been rejected for human consumption.
        2) *Rendering. Rendering* in food processing commonly means separating fat from its connective tissue stroma, or the final treatment of inedible offal (called "tanking"). There are several methods of rendering meat.
            (a) *Dry rendering.* This process, which is generally used for condemned and inedible products, is accomplished with the use of a large horizontal tank surrounded by a steam jacket. The tank contains an agitator that moves the meat about as the fat is separated from other tissue. A partial vacuum allows rendering at a lower temperature. Normally, dry rendering is accomplished at a temperature of about 93.3°C (200°F) in the presence of a partial vacuum. As the meat is processed, it is discharged from the tank into percolating vats where it separates into two layers. The lower layer is the connective tissue residue, usually referred to as cracklings.
            (b) *Wet rendering.* This process is usually employed for removing liquid fat from edible meat. With this method, water is added to the meat after it is placed in the tank. Subsequently, steam is injected into the tank to mix water vapor with the product as it cooks. Finally, the mixture settles out in three layers: the heavy cracklings on the bottom, oil on top, and water between. As the liquid fat is drawn off during cooking, water is injected into the system, causing the remaining fat to rise to the level of the draw-off valves.
            (c) *Centrifuge method.* This rendering process is more complex than the wet or dry methods. It involves continual addition of meat to the system rather than rendering batches. In this method, centrifugal force rather than increased temperature is relied on to separate out liquid fat. Consequently, the process can be accomplished at relatively low temperatures. The meat is ground before centrifuging, enabling easier fat separation during centrifugation. Because of the continuous nature of this process, higher-quality meat must be used. Lower-quality meat requires varying amounts of time to be defatted, which decreases the efficiency of this process. Also, bacterial

contamination is a serious problem with this method. By adding a piece of tissue that is heavily contaminated, considerable amounts of fat can be spoiled. This method is used primarily in operations in which large volumes of meat must be processed rapidly.

b) *Edible products.* Four products can be retrieved from any of the rendering methods described: lard, rendered pork fat, tallow, and oleo stock.

1) *Lard.* This high-quality product is obtained from rendering fresh, clean, normal pork fatty tissue. In other words, fat associated with structures such as bone, skin, or organs may not be labeled as edible lard.

2) *Pork fat.* This edible product can be produced from most tissues but is of somewhat lower quality than lard. A few structures, such as stomachs and headbones, cannot be used. If a whole carcass is passed for cooking, it can be used to produce rendered pork fat. Cured products also can be used for this purpose.

3) *Tallow.* This is simply rendered fat derived from beef and mutton.

4) *Oleo stock.* This product is derived from beef or mutton but differs in that the meat is chilled and hashed before rendering. Rendering in this instance is accomplished in an open tank at about 65.5°C (150°F) as salt and water are added. Oleo stock is the fat that separates out.

c) *Environmental controls.* Several environmental considerations must be reckoned with when rendering inedible products. The objective is simply to prevent cross-contamination of edible products. It is important that separate equipment be utilized. Also, equipment should be well segregated from other processing areas. Personnel who work in this area should have separate clothing for this purpose or do this processing last. In larger operations different employees process edible and inedible products. Odors are controlled most effectively with use of water vapor condensers.

d) *Product controls.* Maintaining the identity of material containing portions of condemned animals is essential. Tanks where inedible products are placed must be sealed to ensure that an inedible product is not retrieved and subsequently processed as human food. In addition, many pathogens can be transmitted via the food chain. Precautions taken to ensure destruction of pathogens minimize the likelihood of their transmission by rendered inedible products used in animal feed.

Salmonellosis outbreaks in the past have occasionally been traced to rendering plants. Because of this, a voluntary *Salmonella*-control program was established under the supervision of Veterinary Services, Animal and Plant Health Inspection Service (APHIS), USDA. The FDA ruled that any animal feed containing salmonellae is contaminated and cannot be sold. The economic implications of the FDA ruling stimulated program participation that probably would not have occurred otherwise. Rendering inedible products usually is not done under strict sanitation.

4. **Poultry Processing**

a) *Essentials in prevention of contamination during processing.* (1) Only healthy poultry should be processed. (2) There should be an abundant supply (numerous taps and large volume) of potable water. (3) Birds with their feathers and feet still attached should be handled in areas separated from areas where evisceration is done. (4) Great care should be taken in removing the digestive organs, in particular the lower gut. (5) Carcasses should be chilled to remove body heat as soon as possible to slow bacterial growth. (6) Personal cleanliness of employees and constant cleaning of equipment should be emphasized.

b) *Processing procedures*

1) *Shipping broilers.* Broilers usually are raised in large houses in large numbers. Often there are 30,000 or more per house. At the end of a 7- to 8-wk growing period, the birds are caught by crews and placed in crates. This process is a potential source of bruising and broken bones. It must be done at night or very early in the morning to avoid piling and overheating. The crates are stacked on trucks for the trip to the slaughterhouse. Cold, very hot, or rainy weather and rough roads may cause losses en route.

Trucks may have to wait at the slaughterhouse to be unloaded. Protective sheds with large ventilating fans are used to prevent losses from overheating or from drenching rain.

While birds are still on the trucks or while the crates are on the unloading dock, an inspector examines the shipment, listening for unusual respiratory sounds and looking for other evidence of sickness. Shipments with a high percentage of sick birds may be rejected and the birds sent back to the farm for treatment.

The birds are taken out of the crates and hung by their legs on a moving line of shackles. This handling is a potential source of bruising and broken bones.

Birds dead on arrival (DOA) should not be hung on the processing line, but through human error dead birds sometimes do go through processing.

2) *Slaughtering.* Humane treatment of animals is increasingly a matter of public concern. Electric stunning of birds is effected as their heads touch a brine solution to complete an electric circuit. Since electric stunning causes high blood pressure, the throat must be cut rapidly to prevent hemorrhages in various parts of the body. This is accomplished using a mechanical throat-cutting device, with a backup worker hand-cutting any birds missed by the machine. Any bird that escapes both must be condemned as a *cadaver,* since it still has all its vessels engorged with blood after drowning in the scalding vat. Its respiratory tract will be full of water and contaminating bacteria.

3) *Defeathering.* Scalding (mild scald at 48.9°C/120°F, hard scald at 57.2°C/135°F) loosens the feathers for picking. The hard scald also removes the outer layer of skin and produces a white-skinned carcass.

After scalding, carcasses enter the rough-picking machine that removes most of the feathers. The setting of the drums (bearing rubber fingers) is very important, since maladjustment may cause skin tears, broken bones, and other damage.

After rough-picking, the birds enter the finishing-picking machine. Feathers missed by the machines are picked by hand. Fine hairlike feathers are removed by passing the birds past banks of flames (called "singeing").

4) *Processing.* The heads of older hens and turkeys must remain attached to the carcass until examined by the inspector. The heads of broilers are removed before inspection. Continuous washing is obligatory. This is near the end of the dirty side of processing.

After these steps have been completed, the lower legs are cut off. It is extremely important that the carcass not be washed after this point (unless the hocks are protected from water) until the inspector observes the carcass to determine if joint exudates are present.

After hock cutting, carcasses pass along a chute and through rubber curtains from the dirty side to the evisceration side of the processing plant. These areas are separated by a wall. Piling up at this point can lead to bacterial decomposition, since the carcasses still have considerable body heat.

After the giblets (heart, liver, and gizzard) are removed, the lungs are removed with a vacuum device, the *lung gun*. The same device is used to remove the ovary from mature hens and the testicles from males. The lungs are likely to contain bacteria that lead to spoilage. Likewise, the yolk material in a mature hen's ovary is a good culture medium and could lead to spoilage if not removed.

After processing, the carcass is immersed in a *chiller* (a large vat in which carcasses are interlayed with crushed ice or a tank with very cold, overflowing water). Rapid chilling is necessary to inhibit bacterial growth. Psychrophilic bacterial populations tend to predominate in such chilled carcasses.

After chilling, the birds are graded and packed. Whole birds are weighed automatically into weight-graded bins and giblets, wrapped tightly in paper, are stuffed into the body cavity. Any carelessness in personal hygiene or in wrapping and placing of the giblets could introduce contaminating bacteria.

Whole birds may be shipped packed in ice or placed in plastic bags and frozen.

Trimmed birds often are cut up into parts. This operation has great potential for buildup of contaminating bacteria, so attention to frequent cleanup of equipment is essential. The various parts are packed in plastic trays overwrapped with plastic and then either frozen or refrigerated. In some operations the air inside the wrapper is replaced with an inert gas to further retard spoilage.

5. **Pasteurization of Milk**
   a) *Pasteurization process.* Pasteurization is defined in the 1978 recommendations of the PHS for Grade A pasteurized milk as follows:

   The terms "pasteurization," "pasteurized," and similar terms shall mean the process of heating every particle of milk or milk product in properly designed and operated equipment, to one of the temperatures given in the following table and held continuously at or above that temperature for at least the corresponding specified time:

Temperature		Time		Common Name
*63°C	(145°F)	30.0	min	Long Time Holding
*72°C	(161°F)	15.0	sec	High Temp, Short Time
89°C	(191°F)	1.0	sec	
90°C	(194°F)	0.5	sec	
94°C	(201°F)	0.1	sec	
96°C	(204°F)	0.05	sec	
100°C	(212°F)	0.01	sec	
138°C	(280°F)	2.0	sec	Ultra-Pasteurized

*If the fat content of the milk product is 10 percent or more, or if it contains added sweeteners, the temperature shall be increased by 3°C (5°F). The term "ultra-pasteurized," when used to describe a dairy product, means that such product shall have been thermally processed at or above 138°C (280°F) for at least 2 sec, either before or after packaging so as to produce a product which has extended shelf life under refrigerated conditions.

The key to success in pasteurization is heating every particle of milk or milk product to the specified temperature and time. The main purpose of the regulations dealing with inspection of pasteurization equipment is to ensure this success.

b) *Purposes.* The purposes of pasteurization are twofold: (1) to destroy any pathogenic microorganisms that might be present in the milk and (2) to enhance the shelf life of milk and milk products.

Although factors such as healthy cows and milk handlers combined with adequate environmental sanitation are important in the production of safe, wholesome milk, pasteurization is still the only effective means of ensuring that pathogenic microorganisms are eliminated from milk without significantly affecting its food value. Pasteurization does destroy some of the vitamin C in milk, but milk is not an important dietary source of vitamin C.

Pasteurization extends shelf life by destroying microorganisms that cause milk to spoil. The process inactivates enzymes in milk that cause deterioration, especially lipase, which breaks down fat to fatty acids, resulting in rancid flavor. Pasteurization is not sterilization. Its purpose is to kill pathogens, not all organisms. Therefore, souring is delayed rather than prevented.

c) *Time-temperature relationship.* Current recommendations for pasteurization are based on the time-temperature requirements (thermal death time) to kill *Coxiella burnetii*, the causative agent of Q fever in man. In 1957, the recommended long-time-holding (LTH) temperature was increased from 61.7° to 62.8°C (143° to 145°F).(See Fig. 1.14)

The previous standard or *pasteurization line* was based on time-temperature requirements to kill *Mycobacterium bovis,* considered earlier to be the most heat-resistant pathogen associated with milk. It was not necessary to change the pasteurization line in the high-temperature short-time (HTST) process as the temperature was sufficient to kill *C. burnetii* and

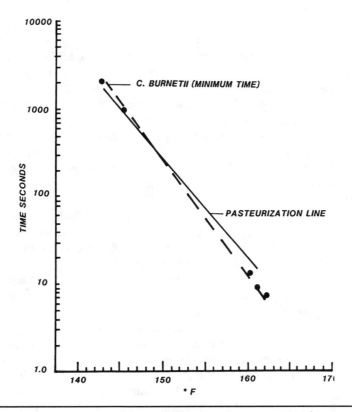

Fig. 1.14. The time-temperature requirements for pasteurization.

M. bovis.

As time-temperature relationships exceed the pasteurization line, the quality of nutritive constituents and flavor of milk is decreased.

d)   *Equipment*

1)   *Pasteurization vat.* A pasteurization vat or tank is used in the LTH method. Adequate agitation is needed so that the temperature of the milk will not differ by more than 1°F (0.56°C) throughout the vat at any time during the holding period.

A milk temperature thermometer is one of three thermometers required on each holding vat. This thermometer also is required on each HTST unit.

To be sure that milk is held in the holding vat for the required time and temperature, a recording thermometer is used. The completed recording charts must be kept for review by the inspector.

The air above the milk in the holding tank must be heated to at least 5°F (2.8°C) above the temperature of the milk to ensure that any milk particles adhering to the side or lid of the tank are pasteurized. This area is heated with an air space heater. The third thermometer measures the temperature in this air space.

2)   *Clarifier.* Clarification is one of the steps done in the plant to prepare

milk for the consumer. Milk is pumped through a centrifugal device, the clarifier, to remove any solid foreign material, particularly blood or somatic cells, straw, or manure. It may be clarified when cold before pasteurization or when hot during the pasteurizing process. The centrifugation isn't sufficient to remove bacteria and has little effect on bacterial count. The clarifier also may be used to separate milk into cream and skimmed milk fractions.

Standardization is done by mixing milk of different butterfat content to prepare a product that meets the butterfat percentage required by law. Inasmuch as the price of milk is determined in part by the butterfat content, standardization is an economic necessity.

3) *HTST unit*

(a) *Flow diversion valve.* In the HTST unit, a flow diversion valve, which is a milk flow stop valve, is installed downstream from the holding tube to prevent forward flow of milk from the holding tube whenever the milk temperature is below 71.7°C (161°F). At such time the valve diverts flow back to the raw milk balance tank. The valve is critical to the HTST process and must be inspected carefully for proper function.

(b) *Holding tube.* Milk is maintained at a specified temperature in the holding tube portion of the HTST unit for a specific period. The tube must have an upward slope of at least 21 mm/cm (1/4 in./ft) from the inlet to the exit to prevent formation of air pockets, which can effectively reduce the holding time.

(c) *Regenerator.* Cold raw milk enters the regenerator section of the HTST pasteurizer from the balance tank. The raw milk is heated by transfer of heat from the already pasteurized milk passing on the other side of the regenerator plate, thereby saving heat. Raw milk in the balance tank must be located so that overflow will be below the lowest level of milk in the regenerator.

(d) *Timing pump.* The timing pump must be located at a point upstream from the regenerator and before the heating section. Milk will thereby be sucked through the regenerator, creating a lower pressure on the raw milk side. If a leak were to occur in the regenerator, the pasteurized milk would flow into the raw milk, not vice versa.

Location of the balance tank below the regenerator also protects against the flow of raw milk past the regenerator should there be a leak in the plate.

(e) *Steam.* If steam is utilized in the pasteurization process, it must be produced from potable water or water supplies acceptable to the regulatory agency and treatment of the water must be as described in the Code of Federal Regulations.

4) *Homogenizer.* Milk is homogenized, usually, by pumping it through a small orifice or other device under high pressure. The fat globules break up to such an extent that after 48 hr of quiescent storage no visible cream separation occurs in the milk. In addition, the fat percentage in the top 100 ml of a quart (0.95 l) differs by no more than 10 percent

from the fat percentage of the remainder after the latter is mixed thoroughly. When homogenization is part of the HTST system, it usually is done between the regenerator section and the heating section or at the end of the holding tube after the flow diversion valve. In the LTH system it is done after preheating to approximately 60°C (140°F) or after pasteurization.

The temperature at the time of homogenization must be sufficient to have inactivated the enzyme lipase to avoid development of hydrolytic rancidity. Homogenization of raw or inadequately heated milk will certainly lead to development of this undesirable rancid flavor.

If the homogenizer is clean and sanitary, no significant increase in bacterial content should occur as a result of homogenization. An increase in bacterial *count* may result, however, because clumps of bacteria are broken up.

After homogenization, the milk is cooled in the same unit in the HTST system or it is pumped to a balance or storage tank (sometimes called a surge tank), from which it flows to a bottling or packaging machine. The milk should be cooled to 3.3°C (38°F) or less before bottling because cooling in the final container is very slow as it depends on air conductivity.

5) *UHT pasteurization*. In the United States the time-temperature relationship for ultra-heat-treated (UHT) milk is 138°C (280°F) for 2 sec. This is achieved either by injecting steam into the milk (which must later be evaporated) or by passing the milk over a plate heat exchanger. This destroys all vegetative forms of microorganisms and most spores thereby producing a much longer shelf life than can be achieved by normal pasteurization. It has the added advantage of minimal flavor change in the milk.

e) *Evaluating effectiveness of pasteurization*
   1) *Salt conductivity test*. A salt conductivity test is used to determine the time milk is exposed in the holding tube of the HTST unit. After electrodes connected to a galvanometer are attached to each end of the holding tube, a salt solution is injected into the tube and the time to flow measured by change of conductivity.
   2) *Phosphatase inactivation curve*. Alkaline phosphatase is one of the enzymes present in milk. The time-temperature relationship needed to inactivate alkaline phosphatase parallels the pasteurization line. Properly pasteurized milk, therefore, will not contain active phosphatase.

   Two tests are in general use to measure inactivation of alkaline phosphatase as an indicator of adequate pasteurization: the rapid field method and the slower but more sensitive photometric method. Either test has the sensitivity to detect 1 part of raw milk in 2000 parts of pasteurized milk. There are several reasons why the phosphatase test may be misinterpreted. For example, the test depends on release of free phenol by enzymatic action. Any free phenol present on laboratory equipment will result in a false-positive test. In another case, chocolate milk and flavoring substances in ice cream contain phenolic compounds that may produce a false-positive test.

The UHT process, usually used with sterilized products, may result in reactivation of phosphatase. Phosphatase is not inactivated completely by this process, and as the product ages, detectable phosphatase activity may return. Reactivation also may be a problem with products with high butterfat such as butter or cream.

f) *Coliform test.* The presence of coliform organisms in pasteurized milk is not an indication of inadequate pasteurization. Instead, it results from contamination of the milk from some source after pasteurization.

g) *Milk products.* The 1978 USPHS recommendations regarding pasteurization of milk products is as follows:

> Milk products which have a higher milkfat content than milk and/or contain added sweeteners shall be heated to at least 65.6°C (150°F), and held continuously at or above this temperature for at least 30 min, or to at least 74.4°C (166°F) and held continuously at or above this temperature for at least 15 sec.

This 5°F increase in pasteurization temperature for products with higher butterfat or added sugar is needed to accomplish the thermal destruction of microorganisms achieved with a lower temperature-time relationship in milk. It is needed because of slower rate of heat penetration through the thicker or more viscous product.

1) *Cheese.* Cheese making is basically a fermentation process in which microorganisms convert lactose or milk sugar to lactic acid. Antibiotics present in milk inhibit fermentation and cause serious economic loss to cheese manufacturers from wasted milk. Antibiotics appear in milk as a result of treating cows orally, parentally, or by intramammary infusion, and as little as 0.05 IU/ml penicillin, 0.05 mg/ml chlortetracycline, or 0.04 g/ml dihydrostreptomycin in milk will inhibit some organisms used in cheese making. If a cow is treated, her milk must not be used for 48 hr or longer after the last treatment to allow sufficient decrease in the level of antibiotic shed in the milk. Some antibiotics require 96 hr. Laws in many states now require that each tanker truckload of milk be certified as antibiotic-free.

Milk may be pasteurized or heated to subpasteurization temperatures to destroy specific microorganisms. Infrequently, a higher temperature is used, but the adverse effect on milk protein reduces yield. In some instances, raw milk is used. Cheese made from raw goat milk is a major source of *Brucella* infection in South America.

Cheese can be an important source of food poisoning caused by the heat-stable enterotoxin produced by some strains of *Staphylococcus aureus*. Milk may be contaminated with staphylococci all along the route to becoming cheese; (1) staphylococci of bovine or human origin may enter the milk during milking, (2) milk may be contaminated from exposure to any unclean equipment used, and (3) risk of exposure to staphylococci of human origin is especially great in the cheese vat. The staphylococci must multiply in large numbers to produce enough enterotoxin to be a hazard. Once the enterotoxin has been produced, it cannot be removed since it is heat-stable. Two points during cheese manufacture that are especially vulnerable to enterotoxin production are (1) holding the milk in vat pasteurizers at a temperature insufficient for pasteurization but adequate for microbial growth and (2) heating the curd to essentially normal body temperature. Acidification that occurs normally during cheese ripening inhibits multiplication of staphlylocci.

2) *Nonfat dried milk (NFDM).* The milk that remains after the cream has been separated is used to manufacture NFDM. To make 1 kg NFDM, 11.2 kg skim milk is required. NFDM contains 94–96 percent solids, 4–5 percent moisture, and 1.25–1.5 percent fat.

If the skim milk used to produce NFDM is of poor quality, the NFDM also will be of poor quality. Staphylococcal enterotoxin present before the milk is dried will maintain its toxicity although the staphylococci are killed. An extensive outbreak of food poisoning has been associated with NFDM that had been condensed in vacuum pans maintained at a temperature that encouraged staphylococcal growth before drying. The milk should be pasteurized before processing.

3) *Ice cream.* Ice cream can be a source of foodborne infection or intoxication, primarily from use of raw or inadequately pasteurized ingredients. Outbreaks of salmonellosis have been traced to raw eggs used in the manufacture of ice cream.

6. Aquatic Animal Processing
a) *Fish*
   1) *Catfish.* A modern catfish-processing plant closely resembles a poultry processing plant. After the fish have been harvested, they are quickly transported to the plant and unloaded into large vats where they are kept alive until processing. Enough vats are available that the harvest from individual farmers can be kept separate for weighing and inspection. Immediately before processing the fish are stunned by an electric current. As each fish is processed, it passes from station-to-station where trained personnel remove fins and heads, eviscerate, skin, and apportion the meat into selected cuts, and wrap. Immediately after wrapping, the fish are frozen.

   2) *Saltwater fish.* Processing of ocean fish is less formalized than catfish processing. This is partly because of the extreme variability in size of the various edible species and partly because of the size of the catch and the local market. In some instances, fish are transported in ice to a central processing facility where the processing is similar to that in a catfish-processing plant. In other situations, the fish are unloaded from boats, where they have been kept in ice, and processed in small plants located near the fishing port. In some instances, preliminary processing is done on the fishing boat. These smaller operations which are labor intensive and sometimes poorly managed, provide increased opportunity for contamination.

b) *Crustaceans and mollusks*
   1) *Crustaceans.* Most crustaceans (lobsters, crabs, and crawfish) are iced and shipped alive to restaurants and retail outlets. Because of the external skeleton, which must be removed for preparing canned or

frozen fillet meat, a great deal of handling and cleaning is necessary in further processing plants. This not only increases the price of the finished products but also increases the opportunity for contamination.

2) *Mollusks.* As is true of crustaceans, most mollusks (clams and oysters) are iced and shipped to restaurants and retail outlets. Consumption of mollusks carries with it an added risk because, in addition to the extreme amount of handling required to prepare them, a large percentage are consumed raw.

C. DETERIORATION OF FOOD

Objectives

1. Differentiate among psychrophilic, mesophilic, and thermophilic bacteria and indicate how each group may be involved in food spoilage.
2. Describe microbial contamination affecting milk quality.
3. Describe how moisture, color, texture, and marbling affect meat quality.
4. Describe the seven microbial actions causing meat-product deterioration.
5. Describe enzymatic changes that can cause meat deterioration.
6. Describe oxidative changes that can cause meat deterioration.
7. Define and describe the physiologic changes producing the following: PSE, PSS, DFD, and dark cutting beef.
8. Describe the microbial and chemical actions causing deterioration of fish and shellfish.

Text

1. **Type of Microorganisms**
   a) *Psychrophilic, mesophilic, thermophilic, and thermoduric.* Bacteria that cause food to spoil are classified in three groups on the basis of temperatures for optimal replication: psychrophilic, mesophilic, and thermophilic. *Thermoduric* bacteria, such as *Streptococcus thermophilus* (which is also thermophilic), can survive *but do not replicate* at high temperatures.
   b) *Optimal-growth temperature ranges.* Psychrophilic bacteria are primarily spoilage bacteria, such as *Pseudomonas putrificiens,* with optimal replication between −1°C and 20°C (30°F and 68°F) and capable of relatively rapid growth at refrigeration temperatures between 2°C and 10°C (35°F and 50°F). The mesophilic group mostly contains pathogens, such as *Staphylococcus aureus,* with optimal growth between 20°C and 45°C (68°F and 113°F). Thermophilic bacteria are primarily spoilage bacteria, such as *Lactobacillus thermophilus,* with optimal growth above 45°C (113°F), though many can grow at 55°C (131°F) or higher.
   c) *Psychrophiles and spoilage.* Psychrophilic bacteria, because of their ability to multiply at low temperatures, are the most important spoilage organisms. Thermophilic bacteria can cause spoilage but under controlled conditions are useful in making certain products. Thermoduric bacteria can cause spoilage if proper temperature is not maintained.

2. **Milk**
   a) *Contamination sources.* The source of microbial contamination of milk may be within the udder; on the surface of the cow, milkers, and other personnel; or in the environment. Spoilage organisms, especially psychrophilic bacteria, are the main cause of high bacterial counts in raw milk.
   b) *Farm equipment.* Improperly cleaned milking equipment or milk storage equipment is the usual source of spoilage organisms. If storage equipment is not properly sealed, milk may be contaminated from aerosols created during feeding, sweeping, or other activities. Adequate daily cleaning and sanitizing of equipment usually prevent high bacterial counts resulting from contaminated equipment.
   c) *Mastitis.* A healthy lactating udder is not a major source of bacterial contamination. However, the udder may be a source of bacterial pathogens if there is a disease process present. Furthermore, the composition of milk from a mastitic udder is altered. Fat, casein, and lactose decrease whereas serum proteins and minerals increase.
   d) *Hygiene.* Clipping the flanks of cows significantly reduces contamination from hair and adhering debris. Careful washing of the teats with a warm sanitizer before each milking reduces the bacterial count.
   e) *Storage temperature.* Storage of milk at a temperature of 4.4°C (40°F) or less is a major factor in retarding bacterial multiplication. The storage life of milk produced under sanitary conditions is significantly longer at lower temperature. Although bacterial growth in heavily contaminated milk is retarded at lower temperatures, shelf life is shortened greatly because many of the contaminants are psychrophilic bacteria that are capable of rapid multiplication at refrigeration temperatures.
   f) *Bacteria in dairy products.* Bacteria in pasteurized dairy products may be from one or more of four sources: raw milk, plant personnel, processing equipment, and the environment within the plant. Thermoduric bacteria present in raw milk can survive pasteurization. It may be impossible to sanitize equipment adequately as a result of flaws in design or deterioration from prolonged use.
   g) *Personnel.* Dairy-processing-plant personnel, either directly or indirectly, are responsible for most contamination present in finished dairy products. Employees may be the source of human pathogens because of poor personal hygiene at work. Of equal importance are employee work habits that determine how effectively equipment is maintained and sanitized, cleanliness of the plant environment, and the effort put forth to prevent contamination from any environmental source.
   h) *Control.* Whenever contamination occurs in a product, corrective measures can be instituted once its source has been identified. The type of bacterial contamination may be an important clue if the organism is known to have any animal (including human) reservoir, is thermoduric, or resides primarily in some other habitat. Systematic sampling at each stage in processing and handling, retracing every step back to the cow if necessary, will reveal the source.

3. **Meat**
    a) *Meat quality*. The term *meat quality* refers to the physical or chemical properties that relate to its processing and palatability characteristics. Four factors are of primary importance in determining the quality of any meat product.
        1) *Water-holding capacity*. The natural moisture content of muscle is approximately 68–78 percent. There are inherent differences in *water-holding capacity* of meats, but generally these are less important than moisture loss during processing and cooking. Excessive moisture lost in processing or through improper cooking will result in a less tender product that is perceived to be poorer in quality.
        2) *Color*. Color can influence the consumer's psychologic perception of quality of a meat product more than actual palatability. Appealing color secondarily influences the retail cost of various cuts. There *is*, of course, a relationship between color and quality; it has been well established that as animals age, the meat becomes darker. Also, surface contamination with microorganisms alters meat color, the color in this instance reflecting a reduction of quality.
        3) *Texture*. Texture of the meat product is determined by feeling and handling the tissue in the uncooked state. Coarse-textured meat is regarded as less tender. Texture is determined by the size of individual muscle fibers and the amount of connective tissue present.
        4) *Marbling*. Marbling (the intramuscular fat) is an important palatability characteristic of meat and is used to determine quality grading of meat. This factor, in addition to moisture-holding ability, is an important influence on flavor among different species. Carbonyl compounds, found in the fat-soluble part of meat, are the major contributors to flavor.
    b) *Causes of meat deterioration*. When efforts to preserve a meat product fail, it deteriorates from one of three causes: microbiologic, enzymatic, or oxidative.
        1) *Microbial changes*. Microbial contamination resulting in deterioration of a meat product usually occurs as the product is handled in the plant. Before death, normal healthy tissue is reasonably free of microorganisms. The number of contaminating organisms that may be present in the carcass depends a great deal on environmental conditions such as the holding temperature, relative humidity, and pH of the product, as well as the inherent characteristics of the meat itself. Under different conditions, we may see seven different microbial changes in meat: acid or gas production, slime formation, mold growth, bacterial greening, formation of green rings, or green cores.
            (a) *Acid production*. Acid production by certain microorganisms often is desirable as a flavor enhancer. In excessive amounts, acids are undesirable.
            (b) *Gas production*. Many microorganisms produce gas. This may be manifested as sausage casings that have burst, meat with a spongy texture, or canned products with swollen lids. Gas production is associated most often with undercooked products or meat products that were not held at a temperature sufficient to destroy the

microorganisms. Gas production indicates the possible occurrence of serious intoxication if the product is ingested. The most serious threat is *Clostridium perfringens*.

(c) *Slime formation*. Slime formation is the result of mass accumulation of microbes on the meat surface. Lactobacilli, micrococci, and yeast most commonly are responsible for this deteriorative change. Contamination of this product results from exposure to personnel or contaminated equipment. These microorganisms grow well at reduced temperatures. Good sanitation is the best means of controlling the problem.

(d) *Mold growth*. Vacuum packaging, which renders the product devoid of oxygen, is a very effective method of combating deterioration by mold. The growth occasionally seen on the surface of products such as dried sausage is not caused by mold, but is rather the result of micrococci or yeast that can survive at a lower humidity.

(e) *Bacterial greening*. Greening of sausages and other cured meats is another microbial change that occurs occasionally in the production of these foods. Bacterial greening results from surface contamination after processing. The microorganisms that cause this change grow readily under aerobic conditions and produce hydrogen peroxide. It is this metabolite that causes greening of the meat. This problem, like other changes that result from microbial contamination, can be prevented by strict hygiene and holding the final product at cold temperatures.

(f) *Green rings*. Green rings, a change that resembles bacterial greening, differ in that they are associated with a heavy population of bacteria in the sausage, etc., before cooking and processing. Strict hygienic measures must be used in processing to prevent the problem.

(g) *Green cores*. Another microbial change in processed meat products, *green cores,* depends on several events occurring in series. First, the sausage emulsion must be heavily inoculated. Subsequently, the processing temperature must be insufficient to kill the microorganisms in the center of the product, that is, less than 68.3°C (155°F). Finally, the finished product must be held at a temperature that enables growth of organisms not destroyed previously. This problem is prevented best by increasing the processing temperature to a minimum of 68.3°C (155°F) as well as by employing good sanitation.

2) *Enzymatic changes*. Two types of enzymes cause changes in meat products: proteinases and lipases. These enzymatic changes are not always undesirable (e.g., enzymes are often used in meat tenderization). If the process is excessive, it is undesirable.

(a) *Proteinases*. Plants are the source of the most common exogenous proteinases, which are used for tenderizing meat: papain, bromelin, and ficin. Fungal proteolytic enzymes, although used in tenderizing, only give a superficial tenderness to a meat product; in other words, they tend to have less penetrability. Inherent proteolytic enzymes, the cathepsins, are very effective in tenderizing meat. Swift and Company has developed an alternative method for tenderizing meat.

Just before stunning, selected animals are injected intravenously with a tenderizing enzyme. The animal must be killed no earlier than 2 min or later than 30 min after this injection. This is a patented process, and the meat from these animals is called Proten meat. Occasionally, an animal will have an allergic-type response to the injection, in which case it must be held for observation for 24 hr and then, if normal, slaughtered in the usual way. Some people are also allergic to this enzyme.

(b) *Lipases*. Oxidative rancidity, another, less desirable enzymatic change, results from lipases acting on the fat producing "free" fatty acids with a bitter-rancid flavor (e.g., butyric acid). Enzymatic reactions are temperature- and pH-dependent. Each enzyme has an optimal range of activity.

3) *Oxidative changes*. Oxidation is a third process that may result in deterioration of meat products. Fat is especially susceptible to this change. Odor, flavor, and color alterations in the product result from its exposure to oxygen. Oxygen absorption in the product is accelerated by light and heat. Unsaturated fats react with oxygen to form double-bonded peroxides. In the presence of light or heat and oxygen, the reaction may be self-perpetuated until the product is fully oxidized. It follows that, if absorption of oxygen can be prevented, meat products can be prevented from deteriorating by oxidation. First, antioxidants or inert gases can be added to retard or prevent oxygen absorption. Second, storing the product away from heat and out of the light is effective. Third, using a wrapper that prevents product exposure to air is helpful. Wrappers that prevent freezer burn do not necessarily prevent oxidation. Therefore, both considerations must be kept in mind when preserving products.

c) *PSE, PSS, DFD, and dark cutting beef*. These four conditions are encountered frequently in the abattoir. Although the actual mechanisms by which the syndromes occur are not firmly established, meat quality is nevertheless influenced by their presence. Each of these syndromes is recognized by the respective color and texture of the meat.

1) *Pale, soft, exudative (PSE) pork*. PSE is a condition seen in pork. It is felt by many investigators that PSE is a manifestation of porcine stress syndrome. In carcasses with signs of this syndrome, fluid actually can be seen exuding from the tissue within minutes after cross sections are made through it. One researcher believes that this condition is associated with selenium and vitamin E deficiency similar to white muscle disease in lambs and that the fluid loss from cells results from antemortem vascular changes. Others believe that the condition is the result of an inherited predisposition that is expressed at postmortem if increased body temperature and acidosis are present.

(a) *Epidemiologic findings about PSE*. PSE has some interesting epidemiologic features. It is seen in about 15–25 percent of all hogs sent to slaughter. Prevalence of the syndrome is associated closely with the season of the year, being higher in the spring and fall. It is felt that the syndrome is more prevalent at these times because of greater fluctuations in ambient temperature. Because it is observed more frequently in related animals, it is believed to be an inherited trait. Although PSE is seen in all breeds, a higher frequency is seen in some breeds and strains, especially the meatier types.

(b) *Factors associated with PSE occurrence.* There is an association among muscle pH, body temperature, and the occurrence of PSE. The speed with which muscle pH drops is also a factor. PSE muscle undergoes rapid postmortem anaerobic glycolysis and results in accumulation of lactic acid. The resulting lowered muscle pH in the presence of undissipated body heat leads to denaturation of the contractile proteins such as myosin and actin. Excitement in these animals not only increases total body heat but also the rate of anaerobic glycolysis, creating the rather unfavorable situation of a more acidotic animal and more body heat that must be dissipated. After cellular proteins are denatured, they lose their water-binding ability. The meat attains a moist appearance and is termed exudative. Since PSE is associated with an elevated body temperature, the meat quality is lowered even more when the animals are sent through the scalding vat. An already elevated temperature is prolonged by this process.

2) *Porcine stress syndrome (PSS).* PSS, another condition that influences pork quality, closely resembles PSE. During the past few years, this condition has been recognized frequently in swine that have been transported. An etiology has not been well defined.

(a) *PSS lesions on necropsy.* PSS swine have muscle changes observable at postmortem, especially large muscle masses such as the longissimus dorsi, gluteus medius, and major muscles of the hind legs. The muscle lesions are essentially the same as those seen in PSE.

(b) *Epidemiologic findings about PSS.* This syndrome is similar to PSE in that there is a higher prevalence in certain breeds such as the Poland China and Hampshire. Stress appears to be the key factor in differentiating PSS and PSE swine. The stress required to initiate clinical signs in PSS-susceptible individuals varies from mild to severe. The syndrome was first recognized in swine found dead after transport. Recently, it has been recognized that signs of PSS may result from mild stress such as moving from one pen to another.

(c) *Clinical signs of PSS.* Clinically, it is difficult to predict which animals will develop PSS. In white pigs, blanched areas of the skin are contrasted with red and purple areas. Under mild stress, some animals have a characteristic quiver in the tail. More severe signs are related to muscle weakness and finally agonal respiratory movements.

(1) *Temperature and blood characteristics.* Both PSS and PSE have been studied extensively in recent years. Three parameters (pH, PCO_2, and PO_2) were measured in PSS- and PSE-susceptible hogs (Poland China) and in PSS- and PSE-nonsusceptible pigs (Chester White). The control groups were maintained at 22°C (72°F). The experimental groups were stressed by exposure to

heat of 45°C (113°F) for 3 min. Blood gas levels were then determined on all groups. The Poland China group was unable to compensate. Consequently, there was an increase in PCO_2 and a concomitant decrease in pH, as well as a dramatic decrease in PO_2. (See Table 1.3.)

(2) *Temperature and respiration rate*. There was also a steady increase in respiratory rate in the susceptible Poland China hogs, indicating inability to adapt to the higher ambient temperature. The Chester Whites were able to adapt to the new environment, as indicated by a rapid drop to normal respiratory rate after 10 min exposure to 45°C (113°F).

(3) *Increased temperature and heart rate*. Heart rate also was recorded in this experiment. Again, the Chester Whites exposed to 45° (113°F) had a temporary rise in rate, which, after a short time, returned to normal. The heart rate of the susceptible Poland China hogs increased progressively to fibrillation and death. (See Fig. 1.15.)

(4) *Adrenal hormone excretion*. A consistent finding in hogs afflicted with PSS is the lowered levels of adrenal hormones. Nonsusceptible Chester White pigs had consistently higher catecholamine excretion than the PSS-susceptible Poland Chinas.

3) *Dark, firm, dry (DFD) pork*. Some pork normally may be darker in color just as some may be extremely pale as a result of the ratio of red muscle cells to white muscle. Most often, however, pork is darker because the cellular pH fails to fall normally. When pH is in the 6.0-6.3 range (instead of 5.5-5.7), muscle fibers become swollen and more tightly packed. Consequently, there is less cell surface to reflect incident light and, hence, a darker color. With the cell tightly packed, the meat then assumes a rather firm consistency. Swine that have been stressed often yield DFD pork. Consequently, it is usually associated with PSS. Swine that have been stressed and recovered have various degrees of glycogen depletion from the muscle cells. During the recovery period, which allows the body to remove excess lactic acid, the pH is elevated as well. The combination of these events leads to DFD.

4) *Dark cutting beef*. Dark cutting beef is another condition encountered in

Table 1.3. Influence of treatment on blood characteristics of hogs

	PCO_2		PO_2		pH	
	Before	After	Before	After	Before	After
Control (22°C)						
Poland China	51	51	36	44	7.4	7.5
Chester White	71	52	38	36	7.4	7.5
Treated (45°C)						
Poland China	54	87	38	7	7.3	6.3
Chester White	63	40	35	42	7.4	7.5

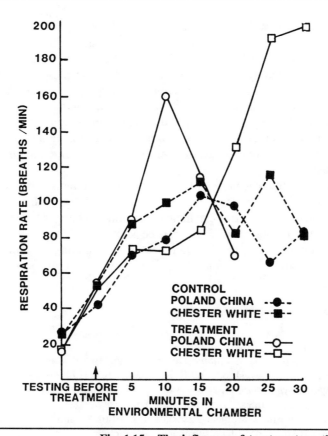

Fig. 1.15. The influence of treatment on the heart rate of hogs.

slaughtering. As the term indicates, it is seen in cattle. The typical history associated with this condition is stress occurring 24-48 hr before slaughter, when for some reason the animal utilized its muscle glycogen stores. Sufficient time elapsed for the excess lactic acid to be removed but not for replenishment of glycogen reserves. Consequently, anaerobic glycolysis is impaired and darker-colored myoglobin predominates. When oxygenated, it is a brighter color (termed *oxymyoglobin*.) The latter form is normally present during life. This condition is seen quite often, but palatability is not impaired. The more expensive cuts (ribs and loins) are affected. It is important commercially because dark cutting beef in vacuum packs tends to "green" as a result of microbial spoilage.

4. **Fish and Shellfish**. Rapid spoilage of fish results from activity of the normal microflora found on the surface and intestinal tract. These organisms survive at 0°C (32°F) and multiply rapidly at temperatures normally used for holding meat and dairy products.

The development of rancidity in fish is the result of oxidation of the oils present in the tissues. Icing, freezing, and salt curing will reduce spoilage during storage, but the oil present in the flesh will undergo deterioration to some extent. In herring stored at 2-4°C (35.6-39.2°F), the acid value (an objective measure of rancidity) doubles in 2 days and quadruples in 6 days.

A direct human health hazard related to improper storage temperature is the development of dangerously high levels of histamine in the flesh of certain scombroid fishes (tuna, bonito, and mackerel) and some non-scromboid fishes (mahi mahi, sardines, anchovies, and herring). The histamine is produced by the action of bacterial decarboxylation enzymes on *histidene,* an amino acid found in these fish.

Shellfish (crustaceans and mollusks) contain far greater amounts of free amino acids than do fish. This facilitates bacterial growth and spoilage. Since shrimp die very soon after catching, deteriorative changes take place earlier than in the other crustaceans, which can be kept alive. The spoilage of mollusks is affected by the presence of certain bacteria: *Pseudomonas, Proteus, Clostridium, Aerobacter,* and *Escherichia* at first and, later, streptococci, lactobacilli, and yeasts.

D. BIBLIOGRAPHY

1. Production

Alexander, J. W. 1963. *Economic Geography.* Englewood Cliffs, N.J.: Prentice-Hall.

Amborski, R. L., M. A. Hood, and R. R. Miller (eds.). 1974. *Proceedings of the Gulf Coast Regional Symposium on Diseases of Aquatic Animals.* Baton Rouge, La.: Center for Wetland Resources, Louisiana State University.

American Veterinary Medical Association Mastitis Committee. 1973. Recommended minimal standards of performance for practicing veterinarians who offer mastitis control programs. *J. Am. Vet. Med. Assoc.* 163:375-77.

Amlacher, E. 1970. *Textbook of Fish Diseases.* Jersey City, N.J.: T.F.H. Publications.

Bardach, J. E., J. H. Ryther, and W. O. McLarney. 1974. *Aquaculture: The Farming and Husbandry of Freshwater and Marine Organisms.* New York: Wiley-Interscience.

Beaujeu-Garnier, J. 1978. *Geography of Populations.* 3d ed. London: Longmans, Green.

Bogue, D. J. 1969. *Principles of Demography.* New York: John Wiley & Sons.

Borgstrom, G. (ed.). 1961. *Fish as Food.* Vol. 1. *Production, Biochemistry and Microbiology.* New York: Academic Press.

_____. 1962. *Fish as Food.* Vol. 2. *Nutrition, Sanitation, and Utilization.* New York: Academic Press.

_____. 1965. *Fish as Food.* Vols. 3 and 4. *Processing,* Parts 1 and 2. New York: Academic Press.

Brown, E. E. (ed.). 1977. *World Fish Farming: Cultivation and Economics.* Westport, Conn.: AVI Publishing.

Chichester, C. O., and H. D. Graham (eds.) 1973. *Microbial Safety of Fishery Products.* New York: Academic Press.

Cole, H. H., and W. H. Garrett (eds.). 1980. *Animal Agriculture.* 2d ed. San Francisco: W. H. Freeman & Co.

Dairy Equipment Testing Co. 1976. Analyzing milking machine performance with the DETCO dual vacuum recorder. Whittier, Calif.

Gregor, H. F. 1963. *Environment and Economic Life.* Toronto: D. Van Nostrand.

Hoffman, G. L. 1974. *Parasites of North American Freshwater Fishes.* Berkeley: University of California Press.

Houser, L. S. (ed.). 1965. *National Shellfish Sanitation Program Manual of Operations. Part 1: Sanitation of Shellfish Growing Areas.* PHS Publ. No. 33, Part 1. Washington, D.C.: U.S. Government Printing Office.

Jensen, E. T. (ed.). 1965. *National Shellfish Sanitation Program Manual of Operations. Part 2: Sanitation of the Harvesting and Processing of Shellfish.* PHS Publ. No. 33, Part 2. Washington, D.C.: U.S. Government Printing Office.

Johnson, S. K. 1975. *Handbook of Shrimp Diseases.* Publ. TAMU SG-75-603. College Station: Texas A&M University.

Jones, G. M. 1975. *Managed Milking Guidelines.* Ext. Div. Publ. No. 633. Blacksburg: Virginia Polytechnic Institute.

Kreuzer, R. (ed.). 1978. *Fish Inspection and Quality Control.* London: Fishing News (Books).

Lovell, R. T., and G. R. Ammerman (eds.). 1974. *Processing Farm-raised Catfish.* South. Coop. Serv. Bull. 193. Auburn: Auburn University.

McDonald, J. S. 1974. Effect of Milking Machine Design and Function on New Intramammary Infection. In *Proceedings, National Mastitis Council Meeting*, pp. 15-39. Arlington, Va.: *National Mastitis Council Meeting.*

Maddux, J. N. 1974. *Milk Rancidity: Causes and Prevention.* Coop. Ext. Serv. Leafl. 199. Athens: University of Georgia.

Mawdesley-Thomas, L. E. (ed.). 1974. *Diseases of Fish.* New York: Academic Press.

Nesheim, M. C. 1979. *Poultry Production.* 12th ed. Philadelphia: Lea & Febiger.

North, M. O. 1984. *Commercial Chicken Production Manual.* 3d ed. Westport, Conn.: AVI Publishing.

Parkhurst, C., and G. J. Mountney. 1987. *Poultry Egg and Meat Production.* New York, N.Y.: Van Nostrand Reinhold.

Poppensiek, G. C., chairman. 1973. *Aquatic Animal Health.* Washington, D.C.: National Academy of Sciences.

Ratcliffe, S. D., and D. S. Wilt (eds.). 1973. *Proceedings of the 7th National Shellfish Sanitation Workshop, Oct. 20-22, 1971.* DHEW Publ. (FDA) 74-2005. Washington, D.C.: U.S. Government Printing Office.

Reichenbach-Klinke, H., and E. Elkan. 1972. *The Principal Diseases of Lower Vertebrates.* New York: Academic Press.

Ribelin, W. E., and G. Migaki (eds.). 1975. *The Pathology of Fishes.* Madison: University of Wisconsin Press.

Roberts, R. J. (ed.). 1978. *Fish Pathology.* London: Bailliere Tindall.

Schalm, O. W., E. J. Carroll, and N. C. Jain. 1971. *Bovine Mastitis.* Philadelphia: Lea & Febiger.

Schultz, W. D., J. W. Smith, and P. D. Thompson (eds.). 1978. *Proceedings of the International Symposium on Machine Milking.* Washington, D.C.: National Mastitis Council.

Sindermann, C. J. 1970. *Principal Diseases of Marine Fish and Shellfish.* New York: Academic Press.

Sindermann, C. J. (ed.). 1974. *Diagnosis and Control of Mariculture Diseases in the United States.* Tech. Ser. Rep. No. 2. Highlands, N.J.: Middle Atlantic Coastal Fisheries Center, National Oceanic and Atmospheric Administration, U.S. Department of Commerce.

Stansby, M. E. (ed.). 1976. *Industrial Fishery Technology.* Huntington, N.Y.: R. E. Krieger.

United Nations. Department of Fisheries. 1972. *Atlas of the Living Resources of the Seas.* Rome: Food and Agriculture Organization.

_____. 1984. *FAO Animal Health Yearbook.* Rome: Food and Agriculture Organization.

_____. Food and Agriculture Organization. 1968. *Fisheries in the Food Economy.* Basic Stud. No. 19. Rome: Food and Agriculture Organization.

_____. World Health Organization. 1974. *Fish and Shellfish Hygiene.* Tech. Rep. Ser. 550. Geneva: World Health Organization.

U.S. Department of Agriculture. 1988. *Agricultural Statistics.* Washington, D.C.: U.S. Government Printing Office.

_____. *Fact Book of U.S. Agriculture.* Misc. Publ. No. 1063. Washington, D.C.: U.S. Government Printing Office.

_____. *1988 Agricultural Chartbook.* Agric. Handb. No. 673. Washington, D.C.: U.S. Government Printing Office.

_____. Agricultural Marketing Service, Livestock Division, Washington, D.C. Livestock, Meat, Wool Market News. Washington, D.C.: U.S. Government Printing Office. (weekly)

_____. Agricultural Research Service, National Cooperative Dairy Herd Improvement Program, Agricultural Research Center West, Beltsville, Md. 20705. Dairy Herd Improvement Letter. (monthly)

_____. Economic Research Service, Commodity Economics Division, Washington, D.C. 20250. Cotton and Wool Situation; Dairy Situation; Fats and Oils Situation; Livestock and Meat Situation; National Food Situation; Poultry and Egg Situation. (periodicals)

_____. Federal-State Market News Service, 801 Badger Rd., Madison, Wis. 53713. Dairy Market News. (weekly)

_____. Federal-State Market News Service, 1718 Peachtree St. N.W., Atlanta, GA. 30309. Egg Report; Poultry Report. (Mon., Wed., Fri.)

_____. Statistical Reporting Service, Crop Reporting Board, Washington, D.C. Cattle on Feed; Eggs, Chickens and Turkeys; Hogs and Pigs; Lamb Crop and Wool; Livestock Slaughter; Meat Animals; Milk Production; Sheep and Goats; Sheep and Lambs on Feed; Wool and Mohair. (periodicals)

U.S. Department of Commerce. *Special Reports 5.* (Dec. 1973).

_____. 1976. *A Marine Fisheries Program for the Nation.* Washington, D.C.

_____. Bureau of the Census. *Census of Agriculture.* Graphic summary, Part 15. Washington, D.C.: U.S. Government Printing Office.

U.S. Department of Health, Education, and Welfare. 1970. *Screening and Confirmatory Tests for the Detection of Abnormal Milk.* Rev. Washington, D.C.: U.S. Government Printing Office.

_____. 1973. *Milk Laboratories Approved by Federal and State Agencies.* Washington, D.C.: U.S. Government Printing Office.

_____. 1971. *Sanitation Ordinance for Condensed and Dry Milk Products Used in Grade A Pasteurized Milk Products.* Washington, D.C.: U.S. Government Printing Office.

_____. 1973. *Procedures Governing the Cooperative State-Public Health Service Program for Certification of Interstate Milk Shippers.* Rev. Washington, D.C.: U.S. Government Printing Office.

_____. 1978. *Grade A Condensed and Dry Milk Products and Condensed and Dry Whey: 1978 Recommendations.* Washington, D.C.: U.S. Government Printing Office.

_____. 1978. *Methods of Making Sanitation Ratings of Milksheds.* Washington, D.C.: U.S. Government Printing Office.

_____. 1978. *Fabrication of Single-Service Containers and Closures for Milk and Milk Products.* Washington, D.C.: U.S. Government Printing Office.

_____. Food and Drug Administration. 1978. *Grade "A" Pasteurized Milk Ordinance, 1978: Recommendations of the United States Public Health Service, Food and Drug Administration.* PHS Publ. No. 229. Washington, D.C.: U.S. Government Printing Office.

University of California, Davis, Agricultural Extension Service. 1967. *Milking Management and Its Relationship to Milk Quality.* Agric. Ext. Serv. Publ. AXT-94. Davis: University of California.

Van Duijn, C. 1973. *Diseases of Fishes*. 3d ed. Springfield, Ill.: Charles C. Thomas.

Wood, P. C. 1976. *Guide to Shellfish Hygiene*. WHO Offset Publ. No. 31. Geneva: World Health Organization.

2. Processing

Arbuckle, W. S. 1977. *Ice Cream*. 3d ed. Westport, Conn.: AVI Publishing.

Beck, J. R. (ed.) 1979. *Vertebrate Pest Control and Management Materials*. ASTM Spec. Tech. Publ. 680. Philadelphia: American Society for Testing and Materials.

Burton, H., J. Pien, and G. Thieulin. 1969. *Milk Sterilization*. FAO Agric. Stud. No. 65. Rome: Food and Agriculture Organization.

Campbell Soup Co. 1975. *Manual of Warehouse Sanitation Guidelines and Sanitation Procedures*. Camden, N.J.: Tech. Admin. Dept., Campbell Soup Co.

Desrosier, N. W. 1977. *The Technology of Food Preservation*. 4th ed. Westport, Conn.: AVI Publishing.

Eckles, C. H., W. B. Combs, and H. Macy. 1951. *Milk and Milk Products*. 4th ed. New York: McGraw-Hill.

Foster, E. M., chairman. 1975. *Prevention of Microbial and Parasitic Hazards Associated with Processed Foods. A Guide for the Food Processor*. Washington, D.C.: National Academy of Sciences.

Fraser, F. M. 1981. Historical overview and potential of food irradiation. Ottawa: Atomic Energy Commission of Canada.

Goldblith, S. A., M. A. Joslyn, and J. T. R. Nickerson. 1961. *Introduction to Thermal Processing of Foods*. Westport, Conn.: AVI Publishing.

Graham-Rack, B., and R. Binstead. 1973. *Hygiene in Food Manufacturing and Handling*. 2d ed. London: Food Trade Press.

Greenberg, A. E. (ed.). 1985. *Standard Methods for the Examination of Water and Wastewater*. 16th ed. Washington, D.C.: American Public Health Association.

Guthrie, R. K. (ed.). 1988. *Food Sanitation*. 3d ed. Westport, Conn.: AVI Publishing.

Hall, C. W., and T. I. Hedrick. 1977. *Drying Milk and Milk Products*. 2d ed. Westport, Conn.: AVI Publishing.

Hall, C. W., and G. M. Trout. 1968. *Milk Pasteurization*. Westport, Conn.: AVI Publishing.

Henderson, J. L. 1971. *The Fluid Milk Industry*. 3d ed. Westport, Conn.: AVI Publishing.

Josephson, E. S., and M. S. Peterson (eds.). 1982. *Preservation of Food by Ionizing Radiation*. Boca Raton, Fla.: CRC Press.

Kosikowski, F. 1982. *Cheese and Fermented Milk Foods*. 3d ed. Ann Arbor, Mich.: Edwards Bros.

Kramlich, W. E., A. M. Pearson, and F. W. Tauber. 1973. *Processed Meats*. Westport, Conn.: AVI Publishing.

Ley, F. V. 1983. New interest in the use of irradiation in the food industry. *Soc. Appl. Bact. Symp. Ser.* 11:113-29.

Libby, J. A. (ed.). 1975. *Meat Hygiene*. 4th ed. Philadelphia: Lea & Febiger.

Longree, K. 1972. *Quantity Food Sanitation*. 2d ed. New York: John Wiley & Sons.

Lowrie, R. (ed.). 1981. *Developments in Meat Science*. Development Series. Barking, Engl.: Applied Science Publishers.

Mann, I. 1960. *Meat Handling in Underdeveloped Countries*. Rome: Food and Agriculture Organization.

_____. 1962. *Processing and Utilization of Animal By-products*. Rome: Food and Agriculture Organization.

Meyer, A. 1973. *Processed Cheese Manufacture*. London: Food Trade Press.

Mitchell, J. R. 1980. *Guide to Meat Inspection in the Tropics*. 2d ed. Farnham Royal,

Bucks, Engl.: Commonwealth Agricultural Bureaux.

Monro, H. A. U. 1969. *Manual of Fumigation for Insect Control.* 2d ed. FAO Agric. Stud. No. 79. Rome: Food and Agriculture Organization.

Mountney, G. J. 1976. *Poultry Products Technology.* 2d ed. Westport, Conn: AVI Publishing.

Mountney, G. J. (ed.). 1987. *Practical Food Microbiology and Technology.* 3d ed. New York, N.Y.: Van Nostrand Reinhold.

North, C. E., and W. H. Park. 1927. Standards for milk pasteurization. *Am. J. Hyg.* 7:147-73.

Palm, C. E., chairman. 1969. *Principles of Plant and Animal Pest Control.* Vol. 3. *Insect-Pest Management and Control.* Publ. 1965. Washington, D.C.: National Academy of Sciences.

Schultz, H. W., E. D. Day, and L. M. Libbey (eds.) 1967. *Symposium on Foods: The Chemistry and Physiology of Flavors.* Westport, Conn.: AVI Publishing.

Skala, J. H., E. L. McGown, and P. P. Waring. 1987. Wholesomeness of irradiated food. *J. Food Protection* 50: 150-60.

Smith, R. F., chairman. 1976. *Pest Control: An Assessment of Present and Alternative Strategies. Vol. 5, Pest Control and Public Health.* Washington, D.C.: National Academy of Sciences.

Stewart, G. F., and J. C. Abbot. 1972. *Marketing Eggs and Poultry.* FAO Mark. Guide No. 4. Rome: Food and Agriculture Organization.

3-A Sanitary Standards Committee. 1978. *3-A Sanitary Standards.* Ames, Iowa: Journal of Food Protection.

United Nations. Food and Agriculture Organization. 1970. *Joint FAO/WHO Expert Committee on Milk Hygiene, Third Report.* FAO Agric. Stud. No. 83. Rome: Food and Agriculture Organization.

United Nations. Food and Agriculture Organization. 1984. *Codex General Standards for Irradiated Food and Recommended International Code for Practice.* Codex Alimentarius XV. Rome: Food and Agriculture Organization.

_____. World Health Organization. 1972. *Vector Control in International Health.* Geneva: World Health Organization.

_____. 1973. *Specifications for Pesticides Used in Public Health.* 4th ed. Geneva: World Health Organization.

_____. 1974. *Equipment for Vector Control.* 2d ed. Geneva: World Health Organization.

U.S. Department of Agriculture. 1973. *U.S. Inspected Meat-packing Plants: A Guide to Construction, Equipment, Layout.* Agric. Handb. No. 191. Washington, D.C.: U.S. Government Printing Office.

_____. Animal and Plant Health Inspection Service. 1972. *List of Chemical Compounds Authorized for Use under USDA Inspection Programs.* Washington, D.C.

_____. Animal and Plant Health Inspection Service. 1979. *Meat and Poultry Inspection Regulations.* Washington, D.C.

U.S. Department of Health, Education and Welfare. Food and Drug Administration. 1975. *Current Concepts in Food Protection.* Cincinnati, Ohio: Cincinnati Training Facility, Food and Drug Administration.

_____. Public Health Service. 1978. *Grade A Pasteurized Milk Ordinance: Recommendations of the United States Public Health Service, Food and Drug Administration.* PHS Publ. No. 229. Washington, D.C.: U.S. Government Printing Office.

Van Arsdel, W. B., M. J. Copley, and A. I. Morgan, Jr. (eds.). 1973. *Food Dehydration.* 2d ed. Vol. 1. *Drying Methods and Phenomena;* Vol. 2, *Practices and Applications.* Westport, Conn.: AVI Publishing.

Webb, B. H., and E. O. Whittier. 1970. *By-products from Milk.* 2d ed. Westport, Conn.: AVI Publishing.

Wilson, A. 1980. *Practical Meat Inspection.* 3d ed. London: Blackwell Scientific Publications.

Wong, N. P. 1988. *Fundamentals of Dairy Chemistry.* 3d ed. Westport, Conn.: AVI Publishing.

Woolrich, W. R., and E. R. Hollowell. 1970. *Cold and Freezer Storage Manual.* Westport, Conn.: AVI Publishing.

3. Deterioration

Defigueiredo, M. P., and D. F. Splittstoesser (eds.) 1976. *Food Microbiology: Public Health and Spoilage Aspects.* Westport, Conn.: AVI Publishing.

Guyton, A. C. 1986. *Textbook of Medical Physiology.* 7th ed. Philadelphia: W. B. Saunders.

Hammer, B. W. 1948. *Dairy Bacteriology.* 3d ed. New York: John Wiley and Sons.

Hausler, W. J., Jr. (ed.) 1974. *Standard Methods for the Examination of Dairy Products.* 13th ed. Washington, D.C.: American Public Health Association.

Jones, T. C., and R. D. Hunt. 1983. *Veterinary Pathology.* 5th ed. Philadelphia: Lea & Febiger.

Libby, A. J. (ed.). 1975. *Meat Hygiene.* 4th ed. Philadelphia: Lea & Febiger.

Pederson, C. S. 1971. *Microbiology of Food Fermentations.* Westport, Conn.: AVI Publishing.

Sharf, J. M. (ed.). 1966. *Recommended Methods for the Microbiological Examination of Foods.* 2d ed. Washington, D.C.: American Public Health Association.

Tanner, F. W. 1944. *The Microbiology of Foods.* 2d ed. Champaign, Ill.: Garrard Press.

2 Foodborne Disease

A. SOURCES OF FOOD CONTAMINATION

Objectives

1. Define primary and secondary sources of food contamination and distinguish between them.
2. Identify sources of primary contamination.
3. Identify sources of secondary contamination.

Text

1. **Types of Sources of Food Contamination.** The source of food contamination may be *primary*, coming directly from an infected food animal or its discharges, or *secondary*, resulting from contamination in handling of food.

2. **Primary Contamination**
   a) *Infected animals.* A food animal may be knowingly or unknowingly sent to slaughter while it is either infected with a microbial agent of disease or contaminated with chemical or other residues. In some instances, this presents an occupational hazard to stockyard or abattoir workers, and it often poses a threat to the health of the consumer. Antemortem inspection reveals only a small percentage of these cases. To cope with this problem, the Food Safety and Inspection Service (FSIS) has incorporated sampling procedures into the USDA inspection program that may be applied to animals before slaughter as well as after.
   b) *Fecal pollution from infected animals.* A second way in which primary contamination may enter the food chain is through the discharges (primarily fecal) of infected animals. Loading a few pigs excreting *Salmonella* into a stock truck with uninfected pigs will result in a high prevalence of new infections after a day's trip to the abattoir. During the slaughtering process,

great care must be taken to prevent fecal contamination of the carcass when the viscera are removed.

3. **Secondary Contamination.** Secondary contamination may come from infected humans, other animals, fomites, or feed additives.
    a) *Infected humans.* Infected humans may be the source of contamination at any point in the food chain but are most frequently implicated in foodborne outbreaks as a result of their activities in the preparation of table food. Loving parents excreting large numbers of staphylococcal organisms,, or restaurant cooks dispensing salmonellae along with the egg salad, have compiled impressive records as sources of food contamination.
    b) *Other animals*
        1) *Vertebrates.* Animals, rodents in particular, are familiar villains in the battle to prevent secondary food contamination. Like humans, their activities may take place at any stage in the food production chain, contaminating stored animal feed on the farmer's premises, raw materials and finished products in the slaughterhouse, or food stored in retail outlets, restaurants, or private homes. In addition to contaminating food with their feces and urine, they are responsible for a staggering amount of food loss on a worldwide basis due to the amount of food they consume.
        2) *Invertebrates.* Invertebrate animals have the dubious distinction of competing with humans for food at every stage of the food chain, right up to the consumer's lips. Because of their diminutive size and vast numbers, they are capable of contaminating food that is safe from larger vermin. For the most part, they pose a threat to the health of consumers by acting as mechanical vectors of disease-producing microorganisms. Like rodents, they exacerbate the problem of an insufficient world food supply. In addition to consumed stored food, they make large quantities of it esthetically unpalatable as a result of their activities.
    c) *Fomites.* Water, soil, plants, and air may serve as vehicles for foodborne disease agents.
        1) *Water.* Because water is used as a cleansing agent in many food-processing steps, it can pose a serious threat to human health if contaminated. One salmonella-infected carcass going through a machine in an abattoir can contaminate the water sufficiently to transmit this disease agent to a large percentage of the carcasses that follow.
        2) *Soil.* Soil is an important vehicle for foodborne disease agents. Depending on the moisture, alkalinity, temperature, and organic material present, soil can support microorganisms for long periods and can serve not only as a source of secondary contamination of food but also as the means for primary contamination by food animals. This contamination may take place not only by ingestion but by other routes such as inhalation of dust, wound contamination, or entry through relaxed teat sphincters.
        3) *Plants.* Plants can serve as a source of food contamination in several ways. Ingestion of wild onions by dairy cows causes the milk from these cows to have a decided off-flavor. Certain toxic plants can remove

animals from the food supply by causing death or a disease condition severe enough to result in condemnation of the animal as unfit for human consumption. Other plants, while not toxic in themselves, can serve as concentrators of environmental pollutants.

4) *Air*. Staphylococcal foodborne disease occurs more often as the result of airborne contamination than from the classic skin pustule or sore. Coughs and sneezes are very efficient ways of disseminating these pathogens, and under normal conditions a person with a good load of staphylococci in the anterior nares can contaminate vast areas in a kitchen or food-processing facility.

d) *Food additives*. Food additives can serve as the source of food contamination in several ways. Addition of a toxic chemical rather than a harmless material may result from carelessness or mislabeling. Utilization of antibiotics as additives in animal-feed supplements also can be a source of food contamination when sufficient withdrawal time is not observed, resulting in unacceptable residue levels.

B. MICROBIOLOGIC CAUSES OF FOODBORNE DISEASE

Objectives

1. Differentiate between foodborne infection and intoxication in microbiologically caused foodborne disease.
2. Describe staphylococcal food poisoning and botulism.
3. Describe the epidemiologic characteristics of foodborne diseases due to bacteria, viruses, fungi, plankton, and parasites.

Text

1. **Foodborne Disease**
    a) *Foodborne disease outbreaks*. Bacteria are the most important cause of foodborne disease. About 75 percent of foodborne outbreaks in the United States are of microbial etiology (Table 2.1).
    b) *Foodborne disease cases*. When the individual cases involved in foodborne outbreaks are tabulated, an even greater preponderance of bacterial etiology is found. Bacteria and viruses are responsible for clinical disease in more than 90 percent of the cases in outbreaks of foodborne disease. Most of the cases reported are caused by *Clostridium perfringens,* salmonellae, and *Staphylococcus aureus* (Table 2.1).
    c) *Foodborne infection vs. foodborne intoxication*. Microorganisms may cause foodborne disease in either of two ways. *Intoxications* involve pathologic changes in the host caused by toxins formed before ingestion. Foodborne *infections,* on the other hand, result from replication of the microorganisms after ingestion.

Table 2.1 Confirmed foodborne disease outbreaks, cases, and deaths, by etiologic agent, United States, 1985

Etiologic Agent	Outbreaks		Cases		Deaths	
	No.	%	No.	%	No.	%
Bacterial						
Bacillus cereus	7	3.2	42	0.2	0	0.0
Brucella	1	0.5	9	0.0	0	0.0
Campylobacter	9	4.1	174	0.8	0	0.0
Clostridium botulinum	17	7.7	33	0.1	2	2.7
C. perfringens	6	2.7	1,016	4.4	0	0.0
Escherichia coli	1	0.5	370	1.6	0	0.0
Salmonella	79	35.9	19,660	85.5	20	26.7
Shigella	6	2.7	241	1.0	0	0.0
Staphylococcus aureus	14	6.4	421	1.8	0	0.0
Streptococcus, group A	1	0.5	12	0.1	0	0.0
Vibrio cholerae	1	0.5	2	0.0	0	0.0
Other bacteria	1	0.5	152	0.7	52	69.3
Total	143	65.0	22,132	96.3	74	98.7
Chemical						
Ciguatoxin	27	12.3	106	0.5	0	0.0
Heavy metals	3	1.4	13	0.1	0	0.0
Mushrooms	1	0.5	4	0.0	0	0.0
Scombrotoxin	15	6.8	57	0.2	0	0.0
Shellfish	2	0.9	3	0.0	0	0.0
Other chemical agents	10	4.5	209	0.9	0	0.0
Total	58	26.4	392	1.7	0	0.0
Parasitic						
Giardia	1	0.5	13	0.1	0	0.0
Trichinella spiralis	8	3.6	39	0.2	1	1.3
Total	9	4.1	52	0.2	1	1.3
Viral						
Hepatitis A	5	2.3	118	0.5	0	0.0
Norwalk virus	4	1.8	179	0.8	0	0.0
Other viral	1	0.5	114	0.5	0	0.0
Total	10	4.5	411	1.8	0	0.0
Confirmed total	220	100.0	22,987	100.0	75	100.0

Source: CDC Surveillance Summaries, March 1990.

2. **Bacteria Commonly Associated with Foodborne Intoxication.** Two foodborne diseases, staphylococcal food poisoning and botulism, are the result of the action of preformed toxins. Intoxications are especially important because, even though a food is prepared so that microorganisms are dead, the preformed toxin may remain if resistant to inactivation (e.g., by heat). Incubation time is important in differentiating foodborne disease associated with ingestion of a preformed toxin from foodborne infections. Preformed toxins may be absorbed by the intestinal tract immediately, whereas infection must await multiplication of the organism

to produce disease.
a) *Staphylococcal toxin*
  1) *Sources and incubation period*. Staphylococcal food poisoning (intoxication) is associated most frequently with coagulase-positive *Staphylococcus aureus*. Staphylococcal organisms are ubiquitous. Most commonly, clinical isolates are from the respiratory tract and the skin (pimples, carbuncles, furuncles, suppurating wounds, etc.) of humans and animals. Food handlers are the most important source of food contamination with these organisms. The incubation period is very short (1–6 hr, usually 2-4 hr). Clinical signs associated with staphylococcal intoxication include nausea, vomiting, diarrhea, and intestinal cramps.
  2) *Foods often involved in staphylococcal poisoning*. Although previous reports have identified ham as the primary vehicle in outbreaks of staphylococcal food poisoning, more recent summaries have indicated a broader range of meats. Beef, chicken, and turkey now vie with ham and other pork products for first place. Salads and pastries with cream filling are other foods frequently implicated.
  3) *Prevention*. Two factors are important in prevention of foodborne outbreaks of staphylococcal intoxication. First, sanitation to prevent contamination, especially by food handlers, must be of paramount concern. Persons with lesions containing purulent exudate should not be permitted to handle food until proper medical advice is sought. Second, outbreaks can be avoided by storing foods at a proper temperature to inhibit growth or destroy the organisms. There is no significant growth at temperatures below 4.4°C (40°F), and the organisms are destroyed when kept at 77°C (170°F) for 20 min. Contaminated food must be maintained at 121°C (212°F) for at least 60 min, however, to destroy the toxin. The latter method is impractical for many foods. Storing foods at temperatures less than 4.4°C (40°F) or greater than 60°C (140°F) effectively prevents (1) *replication of staphylococci* and (2) *significant toxin production*.
b) *Botulinum toxins*
  1) *Types*. Botulism, caused by the toxins *of Cl. botulinum,* is another foodborne intoxication. Several different types of exotoxin are produced by various strains of the organism. Type A is the form encountered most frequently in the United States, whereas in Europe type B is most common. Type E is found in North America, Japan, and Scandinavia. Types C and D affect some animals but not humans. Type F toxin has been identified recently and associated with meat canning in the home. Botulinum toxins are remarkably potent; people have died from merely tasting food that was suspected of being spoiled. These toxins are highly neurotoxic, acting by interference with the synthesis and/or release of acetylcholine at nerve endings. Foodborne, infant, and wound botulism are the three clinical forms.
  2) *Source. Cl. botulinum,* a ubiquitous saprophyte in nature, is a soil resident. It is isolated also from the intestinal tract and contaminated wounds. Although type E is frequently associated with seafoods, it is terrestrial in origin, being carried to the sea, where the spores survive in

the marine environment and are harbored by coastal fish.

3) *Incubation period*. Clinical signs of botulism toxicity are related to action of the toxin at peripheral sites of cholinergic nerves. Although it is an intoxication, it is interesting that the incubation period is often long, ranging from 2 hr to 8 days (average 1–2 days).

4) *Foods commonly associated with botulism outbreaks*. Outbreaks of botulism are commonly associated with certain foods that are canned in the home, such as vegetables and meats. Seafood also has been reported as a source of botulism.

5) *Botulism control in foods*. *Cl. botulinum* is an anaerobic, spore-forming bacillus. Therefore, killing the vegetative organism by cooking is not enough. Canning time-temperature relationships are designed to ensure that *Cl. botulinum* spores are destroyed (121°C/250°F for 20 min destroys spores, 80°C/176°F for 5 min destroys the toxin). The absence of oxygen in canned products is a favorable environment for sporulation and growth of this organism. Therefore, it is important that the organism and its spores be destroyed before the product is canned. Strict sanitation is helpful in preventing the introduction of the organism. In January 1989, the FDA barred interstate shipment of ready-to-eat, salt-cured, air-dried, uneviscerated fish (*kapchunka*) because of the threat of *Cl. botulinum* toxin.

6) *Botulism in babies*. Infant botulism is a form in which botulinal toxin is produced in vivo in the infant gut rather than ingested preformed in food. The clinical spectrum in affected infants extends from mild transient signs of constipation through a more prolonged "failure to thrive" condition to fulminant "sudden infant death syndrome." Almost all cases have occurred in infants 1–6 mo of age. Honey used in infant formula has been a high-risk factor and proven source of *Cl. botulinum* spores.

3. **Bacteria Commonly Associated with Foodborne Infection**. Many foodborne diseases result from infections. Organisms most commonly reported in outbreaks of foodborne infections are *Cl. perfringens, Campylobacter jejuni*, and the *Salmonella* group.

a) *Clostridium perfringens*

1) *Characteristics*. *Cl. perfringens* is a ubiquitous anaerobic spore former. Meat and poultry are associated most commonly with foodborne outbreaks of this disease. Spores often survive the cooking process; when the meat product is later taken from the refrigerator and allowed to stand at room temperature, sporulation and subsequent multiplication of organisms occur in the absence of air. The incubation period is 8–22 hr (average 12–14 hr). Clinical signs, which persist for 8–12 hr, usually involve abdominal cramps and watery diarrhea.

2) *Transmission*. Transmission of *Cl. perfringens* is virtually impossible to prevent because this organism is ubiquitous. It is a common inhabitant of the intestinal tract of humans and animals. Food, therefore, can be contaminated from either source. If the abattoir worker is not hygienic, meat could be contaminated either from the animal or from the worker.

It is also possible for the organism to be introduced into food by unhygienic food handlers. Foodborne outbreaks due to *Cl. perfringens* occur primarily in institutions or commercial food operations where many people handle a food product before it is served and where larger quantities (e.g., big roasts) are prepared.

3) *Control*. Although *Cl. perfringens* spores are usually destroyed when the medium is kept at a temperature of 100°C (212°F) for 30 min, this time-temperature relationship often may destroy the esthetic quality of the food. The basis for controlling foodborne outbreaks is the general rule: Keep hot things hot and cold things cold. That is, to prevent replication, cooked foods should not be held at temperatures between 4.4°C (40°F) and 60°C (140°F).

b) *Salmonellae*

1) *Salmonella serotypes*. There are over 1600 *Salmonella* serotypes. *S. typhimurium* is the most common serotype associated with human salmonellosis, followed by *S. enteritidis* and *S. heidelberg* (Table 2.2).

2) *Nonhuman sources*. Nonhuman reservoirs are an important source of salmonellae for human foodborne disease (Table 2.3). Salmonellae were isolated from 72% of rendered animal feeds sampled by FSIS during a study conducted in 1986. During the same year Agriculture Canada reported finding salmonellae in 10.4% of 318 pork carcasses and 2.4% of 321 beef carcasses. The results of testing broiler chickens, since 1979, indicated the presence of salmonellae in 55% of birds tested. These birds arrive at slaughter plants with the organisms firmly attached to the skin. *Salmonella enteritidis* contamination of eggs has been of major concern as a potential source of human illness.

Table 2.2. *Salmonella* **serotypes most frequently isolated from humans, United States, 1984–1986**

	Number of Isolates						Rank		
	1984	%	1985	%	1986	%	1984	1985	1986
S. typhimurium[a]	12,724	(35)	28,154	(50)	10,888	(26)	1	1	1
S. enteritidis	3,709	(10)	5,611	(10)	5,967	(14)	2	2	2
S. heidelberg	3,575	(10)	5,196	(9)	5,595	(13)	3	3	3
S. newport	1,615	(4)	2,452	(4)	2,431	(6)	4	4	4
S. infantis	1,234	(3)	1,106	(2)	1,104	(3)	5	7	6
S. agona	942	(3)	1,193	(2)	912	(2)	6	6	7
S. saint paul	654	(2)	442	(1)	558	(1)	7	13	11
S. montevideo	637	(2)	715	(1)	775	(2)	8	8	8
S. muenchen	525	(1)	586	(1)	694	(2)	9	9	9
S. oranienburg	502	(1)	501	(1)	484	(1)	10	10	14
S. braenderup	414	(1)	334	(1)	616	(1)	13	15	10
S. hadar	262	(1)	1,197	(2)	1,552	(4)	18	5	5
Subtotal	26,793	(74)	47,487	(84)	31,576	(75)			
Other	9,268	(26)	9,263	(16)	10,452	(25)			
Total	36,061	(100)	56,750	(100)	42,028	(100)			

[a]Includes *S. typhimurium* var. *copenhagen*.

Table 2.3. *Salmonella* serotypes identified most frequently from animal and related sources during fiscal year 1985 with comparison data for 5 years, United States

Serotype	1985		1984		1983		1982		1981		1980	
S. typhimurium	682[a]	(1)[b]	809	(1)	958	(1)	981	(1)	844	(1)	790	(1)
S. cholerasuis var. kunzendorf	559	(2)	562	(2)	592	(2)	621	(2)	611	(2)	706	(2)
S. heidelberg	368	(3)	399	(3)	380	(3)	234	(5)	214	(5)	321	(4)
S. typhimurium var. copenhagen	292	(4)	309	(4)	377	(4)	433	(3)	579	(3)	380	(3)
S. arizonae[c] 18:Z4, Z32	240	(5)	273	(5)	311		224		135		82	
S. anatum	195	(6)	170	(9)	175	(6)	236	(4)	191	(6)	179	(7)
S. montevideo	176	(7)	183	(8)	122	(10)	127	(11)	117	(10)	61	(13)
S. agona	173	(8)	217	(6)	198	(5)	157	(9)	158	(7)	203	(5)
S. sandiego	173	(8)	60	(19)	164	(7)	141	(10)	52	(16)	48	(14)
S. saint-paul	154	(9)	83	(14)	95	(13)	223	(6)	117	(10)	119	(9)
S. dublin	140	(10)	208	(7)	136	(9)	198	(7)	246	(4)	197	(6)

[a]Number of times serotype was identified.
[b]Rank, beginning with the most common.
[c]First included in this table FY 1984.

3) *Characteristics of salmonellosis.* A wide variety of foods are involved in outbreaks of salmonellosis; patients typically have a history of ingesting foods such as poultry, meats, gravies, eggs, fish, shellfish, or milk. Clinical signs include abdominal cramps, diarrhea, vomiting, chills, and fever, accompanied by low case-fatality rates. Illness usually begins in less than 72 hr (average 12-14 hr) after ingesting contaminated foods.

4) *Control.* Controlling and preventing outbreaks of foodborne disease caused by salmonellae involve three general approaches: breaking the cycle, educating the public, and preventing contamination.

(a) *Breaking the cycle.* An important aspect of breaking the cycle involves controlling rendering (separating fat from tissue mechanically or with heat or both, to produce lard, animal feed, and fertilizer) so that animal feeds containing animal by-products are free of viable salmonellae. Shortening the interval between an animal's leaving the farm and its slaughter is helpful in breaking the cycle because environmental buildup of organisms from infected animals will be less and the consequent contamination of stockyards and abattoirs will be less likely.

(b) *Public education.* Public awareness of how *Salmonella* organisms are transmitted is vital to an effective control program. Education should also be concerned with the proper handling and preparation of foods in the home.

(c) *Preventing contamination.* Consumers must be aware that a cooked product can be recontaminated when handled improperly (for example, if a knife and cutting board are not cleaned before they are used for another food after the homemaker cuts up raw chicken or steak, cross-contamination may occur). Foods should be thawed under refrigeration and not exposed to the air because holding foods at room temperature allows for microbial buildup in contaminated foods and, if the foods are left uncovered, possible airborne contamination. Because food handlers may be carriers of *Salmonella* organisms, it is wise to have employees who handle food examined periodically by a physician.

5) *Typhoid*. Typhoid fever is a nonzoonotic foodborne disease syndrome caused by the serotype *S. typhi*. The case of Typhoid Mary is perhaps one of the most dramatic illustrations of the potential danger associated with transmission of infectious agents through the food chain. (There is an excellent account of this case in *Eleven Blue Men*, by Berton Roueche.) This disease has a relatively long incubation period (2-3 wk), and carriers of this organism may shed it intermittently. Because of the insidious nature of this disease, control of outbreaks is difficult. Infected individuals show clinical signs that are often quite vague. Typhoid fever is suspected in patients with anorexia, headache, fever, and diarrhea, especially if the onset of signs and symptoms is slow.

c) *Campylobacter jejuni*. This organism, previously identified as *Vibrio fetus* subspecies *jejuni*, has only recently been recognized as a major cause of foodborne disease. Failure to realize its significance has been largely due to its optimum growth requirements, which caused it to be missed in routine isolation procedures.

1) *The organism*. *Campylobacter* is a gram-negative, microaerophilic, thermophilic organism that grows best at a temperature of 43°C (109.4°F) and requires special media for cultivation. Currently, there are nine named or proposed species that may be pathogenic to humans (Table 2.4). Refrigeration of contaminated foods will promote survival, and freezing may allow long-time survival of a small percentage from an initial large population. Because of its pathogenicity (only 500 cells may produce clinical disease) and wide distribution in nature, it is a leading cause of foodborne disease.

2) *The disease*. The usual incubation period is 3-5 days. Clinical signs include fever, profuse diarrhea (sometimes bloody), abdominal pain, and nausea. The disease usually lasts for 3 days, but illness may reoccur for

Table 2.4. *Campylobacter* species pathogenic or potentially pathogenic in humans

Current Name	Previous Names
C. jejuni	*C. fetus* subsp. *jejuni;* related *Vibrio*
C. coli	
C. laridis	Nalidixic acid-resistant thermophilic *Campylobacter*
C. fetus ssp. *fetus*	*C. fetus* subsp. *intestinalis; Vibrio fetus*
C. hypointestinalis	
"*C. cinaedi*"[a]	*Campylobacter*-like organism-1A[b]
"*C. fennelliae*"[a]	*Campylobacter*-like organism-2
"*C. upsaliensis*"[a]	Catalase-negative or weak strains
C. pylori	*C. pyloridis;* gastric *Campylobacter*-like organisms

[a]Proposed species names.

[b]A separate and unnamed species, *Campylobacter*-like organism-1B, can be distinguished from *Campylobacter*-like organism-1A by DNA hybridization studies, but it is biochemically indistinguishable from "*C. cinaedi*."

periods up to 2 wk. Isolation rates of *C. jejuni* from humans are highest during the first year of life, followed by a second peak during young adulthood, and are slightly higher among males than among females during the first 45 yr of life (Fig. 2.1).

3) *Reservoir.* *C. jejuni* is ubiquitous in foods of animal origin. Poultry is the predominant source with contamination rates of raw poultry products reaching nearly 90% in some studies. Most clinically healthy poultry, swine, and cattle excrete *C. jejuni* in their feces and more than 10^6 cells may be present per gram of feces.

4) *Transmission.* Most outbreaks in the United States have been traced to raw milk, but the organism has been isolated from water and meat as well. Poultry is currently acknowledged as the predominant source. Immature companion animals represent a source of infection, particularly for children. Person-to-person transmission can occur, but as evidenced by reports from day care centers or mental institutions, where person-to-person transmission of infectious organisms is common, it is not usual.

5) *Control.* Mandatory pasteurization of all milk and proper treatment of all drinking water would prevent a large percentage of human campylobacteriosis cases but would do little to reduce the threat from other sources. Proper production, processing, and preparation of foods of animal origin will reduce the level of contamination, but since the organism is so ubiquitous, proper cooking is the only practical control procedure at the present time. It should be noted that microwave

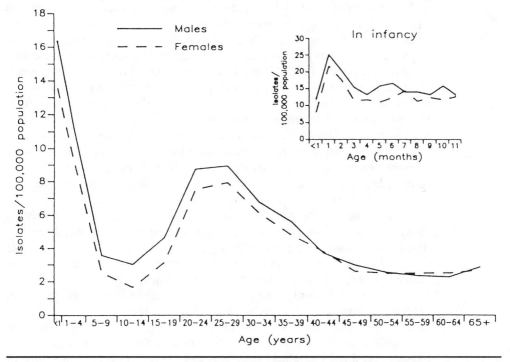

Fig. 2.1. Annual isolation rates of *Campylobacter*, by age and sex, in the United States, 1982–1986.

cooking may not completely remove contamination from meat.

Growing interest has been focused on low-level irradiation as an effective technique for killing *C. jejuni,* particularly in cut-up poultry. This procedure, when coupled with modern impervious packaging techniques, may provide a commercially acceptable method for supplying consumers with a *C. jejuni*-free product.

d) *Streptococcus faecalis.* This microorganism, which commonly inhabits the intestinal tract of humans and animals, is often associated with foodborne disease when it is spread through vehicles such as beef and pork meat products. Signs of infection are milder than those associated with salmonellosis. A person in a typical case may suffer from vomiting, diarrhea, fever, and chills. Typically, the incubation period ranges from 2 to 18 hr. Strict sanitation is the only practical means of controlling this foodborne disease because the agent is fairly resistant to heat treatment, being able to withstand 60°C (140°F) for 30 min.

e) *Hemolytic streptococci.* Hemolytic streptococci inhabit the oropharyngeal and nasal cavities of some individuals. Milk and other foods become contaminated when infected individuals create an aerosol by coughing and sneezing. Mastitic cows also may transmit hemolytic streptococci through milk and cause the typical strep throat syndrome. Usually the incubation period is 3 days.

f) *Bacillus cereus.* This aerobic, spore-forming microorganism, a saprophytic gram-positive rod, has been associated with outbreaks of foodborne disease for more than a quarter of a century. It is isolated with ease from soil, water, and most types of vegetation. Foodborne disease outbreaks are encountered when excessively high numbers are present in food because of poor sanitation or improper handling. The signs, which are similar to *Cl. perfringens* infections but much milder, include nausea and severe abdominal cramps that persist for 6-12 hr. The incubation period is 8-16 hr. Foods involved most frequently in these outbreaks include vanilla pudding, cream sauces, barbecued chicken, and turkey loaf. Control measures are essentially the same as for *Cl. perfringens* infections.

g) *Shigella sonnei.* Shigellosis is another disease that may be foodborne as a result of unsanitary practices. Most cases in the United States are caused by *S. sonnei.* Outbreaks of this disease are a problem in nurseries and day-care centers, because fecal-oral transmission is common among young children. In the United States, the highest incidence of disease caused by shigellae is in young children not yet toilet-trained. Many cases have been seen in monkeys and their handlers. A 1- to 3-day incubation period usually follows direct transmission. The outstanding signs associated with *Shigella* infections include bloody diarrhea and a persistent fever, especially in untreated patients. A carefully taken history or inspection of premises often reveals ingestion of feces-contaminated water, vegetables, or dairy products. Effective control methods involve strict sanitary practices.

h) *Brucella spp.* Brucellosis (human undulant fever) frequently results from transmission of the agent through the food chain, through ingestion of unpasteurized dairy products (meat has not been proved to be a source of infection). An effective control program in the United States has produced a 10-fold reduction in the number of human cases resulting from occupational as well as foodborne exposure over the past quarter century (Fig. 2.2).

Foodborne brucellosis is almost exclusively the result of ingestion of raw milk or raw milk products. Brucellosis is primarily an occupational disease. High-risk groups include farmers, veterinarians, and abattoir workers (Table 2.5).

The incubation period ranges from 3 to 21 days, but it may be several months before clinical signs occur. The recurrent nature of the signs, especially fever, gave rise to the term *undulant fever.*

i) *Francisella tularensis.* Tularemia, occasionally a foodborne disease, is associated with wild game such as rabbits, squirrels, and raccoons. It is contracted more frequently as a result of handling and dressing game than

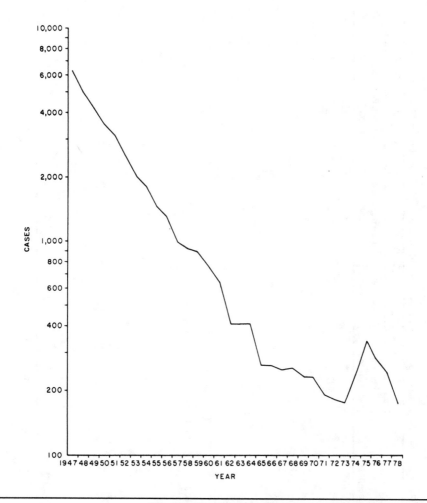

Fig. 2.2. Human brucellosis in the United States, 1947–1978. (CDC Human Brucellosis Surveillance 1978)

Table 2.5. Cases of brucellosis by occupation and most probable source of infection, United States, 1978

Cases of Brucellosis	Meat-processing Industry			Livestock Industry			Other	Unknown	Total	Percent of Total
	Packinghouse employee	Government inspector	Rendering-Plant employee	Livestock-market employee	Livestock producer	Veterinarian				
Domestic animals										
Cattle	12	6	3	2	20	3	4	4	54	33.5
Swine	9	1			4			2	16	9.9
Cattle or swine	10	2	5						18	11.2
Swine, cattle, sheep, or goats					1	1	1	1	3	1.9
Unspecified farm animals	9	1		1		1			12	7.5
Dogs								3	3	1.9
Wild animals										
Feral swine							2		2	1.2
Caribou								1	1	0.6
Unpasteurized dairy products										
Domestic					5		3	1	9	5.6
Foreign					1		3	1	5	3.1
Accidents										
Strain 19 vaccine						3			3	1.9
Laboratory							2		2	1.2
Unknown						1	10	21	32	20.5
Total	40	10	8	3	31	9	25	34	160	100.00
Percentage of Total	24.8	6.2	5.0	1.9	19.9	5.6	15.5	21.1	100	

Source: CDC Brucellosis Surveillance, 1978 Annual Summary.
Note: 160 cases are included in this survey.

through ingestion of infected meat. The incubation period is 8–24 hr. Signs and symptoms include headache, chills, fever, vomiting, and lymphadenitis. Strict hygienic habits while handling small game animals aid in preventing infection. Cooking the meat for 10 min at 57°C (135°F) prevents foodborne transmission.

j) *Vibrio cholera.* The disease agent *V. cholera* is shed from the body primarily in the feces. In endemic areas with poor food hygiene, contaminated food perpetuates the cycle of transmission. Foods commonly associated with cholera outbreaks are vegetables, fish, and pork products. Sewage (night soil) is used commonly to fertilize vegetable gardens in some societies. Sewage contamination of drinking water is a major cause of cholera outbreaks. The incubation period is 2–3 days. Clinical signs include profuse diarrhea with abdominal pain, vomiting, headache, and fever. Death is usually the result of the profound dehydration that accompanies clinical illness.

V. *cholera* 01 has been found along the U.S. Gulf Coast since 1973 and has been incriminated in some cases. Non-01 *V. cholera* is often found in U.S. coastal waters. It can cause diarrheal disease and extraintestinal infections but does not pose the same epidemic threat as *V. cholera* serogroup 01. In the United States, outbreaks are usually caused by eating raw or improperly cooked seafood.

In 1988, a related organism, *V. vulnificus,* perhaps the most virulent of the marine vibrios, was incriminated in 45 cases in that resulted in 17 deaths. Eleven of these fatalities were related to ingestion of raw oysters. As is true of *V. cholera,* this organism can also produce serious wound infections.

k) *Vibrio parahaemolyticus*

  1) *Source.* This organism is commonly associated with seafood and has been isolated from virtually every type of shellfish consumed by humans. Although infections have caused death of certain shellfish, *V. parahaemolyticus* is considered a member of the normal flora.

  Outbreaks of food poisoning result from consumption of high doses (100,000 organisms) in raw, improperly cooked, and/or improperly handled seafood. Clinical signs and symptoms in humans are evident primarily as enteric disease. The incubation period ranges from 4 hr to 14 days (average 12–14 hr). The course of clinical illness often is about 3 days.

  2) *Control.* Control of *V. parahaemolyticus* is fairly simple. Currently, no spread of infection has been recognized from human to human. In areas where raw seafood is consumed, special emphasis must be placed on proper handling and storage. The organism is sensitive to environmental alterations (refrigeration, freezing, and heat.) If products are cooked, thorough penetration of heat >55°C (>131°F) is necessary. In addition, seafood should not be held without refrigeration for extended periods after it is cooked. Outbreaks of *V. parahaemolyticus* infection have occurred as a result of shrimp and crab "boils," when the batches of shrimp or other shellfish were too large to be boiled at once; the shellfish in the center of the cooker were not cooked adequately, allowing organisms to survive and produce foodborne disease.

l) *Yersinia enterocolitica.* Diarrhea, fever, and abdominal pain, usually persisting for several days, are typical of *Y. enterocolitica* infection. In some areas, the frequency of yersiniosis is second only to salmonellosis. Sources of human infection are similar to *C. jejuni*, with swine serving as the main reservoir. Although outbreaks of enteric disease caused by pasteurized milk are rare, the ability of *Y. enterocolitica* to grow at refrigeration temperatures makes pasteurized milk a potential vehicle if contaminated. Control is similar to *C. jejuni*.

m) *Listeria monocytogenes.* Listeriosis, and its association with ensilage, has long been familiar to veterinarians as "circling disease" and a cause of abortion. More recently it has attracted attention as a serious human foodborne disease associated with meningitis, septicemia, and abortion. Approximately 1700 cases a year, with a 25% case-fatality rate, are currently reported.

1) *Source. L. monocytogenes* is a non-spore-forming, motile, gram-positive bacillus that is widespread in the environment and has been isolated from most foods of animal origin. There are at least 11 serotypes, three of which (1a, 1b, and 4b) cause 90% of human clinical infections. The organism is carried asymptomatically in the human intestinal tract of up to 5 percent of the population.

2) *Epidemiology.* The epidemiology of foodborne listeriosis is poorly understood. The incubation period and minimum infective dose are uncertain. The organism has been isolated from meat, poultry, seafood, milk, and milk products and is commonly associated with outbreaks of human illness, but isolation of the organism from suspected foods has been difficult.

3) *Control.* Reduction of outbreaks has been difficult to achieve because of lack of knowledge about the organism. Available evidence indicates that it can multiply and survive for long periods in refrigerated foods and may even increase in virulence at these low temperatures; at the other extreme, it can survive temperatures used in some pasteurization and food processing procedures. At the present time the FSIS, FDA, and CDC are conducting sampling programs at various points in the food processing chain but controversy exists regarding the preferred methodology. Processing plants from which positive samples are isolated at the retail level must recall those products.

n) *Escherichia coli.* Four types of *E. coli* are known to produce gastroenteritis in humans; enteropathogenic *E. coli* (EPEC), enteroinvasive *E. coli* (EIEC), enterotoxigenic *E. coli* (ETEC), and hemorrhagic *E. coli* (HEC). Among these, the first 3 are spread by infected humans, only hemorrhagic *E. coli* has been demonstrated to have a reservoir in animals. Several outbreaks, in which *E. coli* 0157:H7 was isolated from ill humans, have been associated with consumption of rare ground meat and raw milk.

4. **Viral and Rickettsial Organisms Commonly Associated with Foodborne Infections**

a) *Infectious hepatitis virus.* Type A or infectious viral hepatitis of humans is differentiated from type B (serum) hepatitis on the basis of incubation period and other features. The incubation period for type A is 15–50 days, for type B 2–6 mo. Signs and symptoms for either type include fever, jaundice, anorexia, gastrointestinal irritation, and a low case-fatality rate. Type A has been contracted through foods such as dairy products, shellfish, and homemade bakery items (actually, any food unhygienically prepared may be a source of infection). Water is also an important vehicle for transmitting the agent. It is almost always associated with poor personal hygiene and poor sanitation.

b) *Poliomyelitis enterovirus.* Poliomyelitis is potentially a foodborne disease. Raw milk or unsanitary handling of pasteurized milk has been suspected in some polio outbreaks. Several attempts to infect bovine mammary glands have resulted in failure, which indicates that the cow is an unlikely source. Numerous attempts to isolate polio virus from dairy products have also been futile. The most plausible explanation of foodborne disease caused by polio virus is contamination by infected persons.

c) *Enteric cytopathogenic human orphan (ECHO) viruses.* Several enteroviruses, termed the ECHO group, cause gastrointestinal symptoms. It is felt that ECHO viruses are responsible for a significant portion of reported gastrointestinal diseases of unknown etiology.

d) *Norwalk virus.* This calicivirus-like agent was first implicated as the cause of a disease outbreak in Norwalk, Ohio. This agent was responsible for nearly half of all foodborne disease cases reported to the Center for Disease Control (CDC) in 1982, even though associated with only two outbreaks, an indication of its infectivity given the proper conditions. Several serotypes have been identified, resulting in a situation similar to influenza, in which practical immunity is limited. Both foodborne and waterborne transmission can occur via the fecal-oral route.

e) *Coxiella burnetti.* This organism causes Q fever, which is widely distributed in the world. Reservoirs include cattle, sheep, and goats. Transmission occurs primarily by inhalation of infectious organisms, resulting in signs of respiratory disease. The incubation period is 2–3 wk. The food chain also represents a means of transmission; as most milk is pasteurized in the United States, however, food transmission is of lesser importance in this country. Infected animals may shed *C. burnetti* in the milk for long periods (200 days reported).

5. Fungal Organisms Associated with Foodborne Disease

a) *Ergot fungus.* Ergotism is a mycotoxicosis resulting from a toxin-producing fungus that grows on cereal grains such as wheat and rye. A heat-stable toxin is produced that is not denatured by baking or cooking. In the United States, all grains to be used for flour are treated first to prevent toxin production; thus ergotism rarely occurs here. Illness is related to ingestion of the toxin.

b) *Poisonous mushrooms.* This form of foodborne disease can be prevented by not eating poisonous mushrooms. Careful differentiation between edible and toxic types is essential.

c) *Aspergillus spp.* Some strains of *Aspergillus* spp. produce aflatoxin, hepato-toxins that cause disease in animals, including humans. The most common sources have been peanuts, cottonseed meal, corn, and various grains. Suspected foods can be analyzed for the presence of aflatoxin by laboratory procedures.

6. **Plankton Associated with Foodborne Disease.** Foodborne disease also is associated with *plankton* (free-living microorganisms in water). Plankton serve as a food resource for aquatic animals eaten by humans.

   a) *Dinoflagellate toxicity* (paralytic shellfish poisoning). Dinoflagellates and other photosynthesizing organisms are the primary nutrient, either directly or indirectly, of almost all marine life. Under certain conditions these organisms multiply tremendously, resulting in an accumulation of millions of dinoflagellates at the sea surface. These "blooms" vary from white to red (the "red tide") and are followed by increased marine and human morbidity. Some species, primarily members of the *Gonyaulax* and *Gymnodinium* genera, produce a potent heat-stable alkaloid toxin (saxitoxin) that affects vertebrates. Mortality will ensue among fish that consume these dinoflagellates (and among predator fish and birds that eat these fish), but humans are spared because they do not harvest dead fish. Molluscs, however, are not affected by the toxin and are particularly dangerous to humans because they can accumulate levels of these toxins high enough so that a single shellfish may contain a fatal dose. Clinical signs include prickly sensations of the eyes, tongue, and fingertips followed by numbness. Muscular incoordination, an ascending paralysis and death from respiratory failure may follow in 2–12 hr. If one survives 24 hr, the prognosis is good.

   b) *Clinical signs.* Four clinical forms of intoxication occur as a result of exposure: (1) paralytic, (2) erythematous, (3) gastrointestinal, and (4) respiratory. In humans, symptoms of the paralytic form occur usually within 30 min after ingestion of toxic shellfish. Symptoms generally are related to neuromuscular dysfunction. Nausea, vomiting, diarrhea, and abdominal discomfort are associated with the gastrointestinal form. The erythematous form, an allergic reaction, results after an incubation period of a few hours. Occasionally, respiratory irritation occurs among humans during severe red tide episodes, presumably the result of dinoflagellate toxin.

7. **Parasites Associated with Foodborne Disease.**

   a) *Taenia spp.* The adult stages, of two cyclophyllidian tapeworms, *T. saginata* and *T. solium,* parasitize the small intestines of humans. The larval stage (cysticerci) of these parasites occurs in meat from cattle (a condition called beef measles) and swine (pork measles), respectively. (See Figs. 2.3. and 2.4)

      1) *Taenia saginata. T. saginata,* the beef tapeworm of humans, is one of the largest cestodes, with an average length of 5–10 m. Cattle become infected when their feed or pastures are contaminated with feces of humans infected with *T. saginata.* Eggs swallowed by cattle hatch in the duodenum and liberated onchospheres that enter the lymphatics or blood vessels of the hepatic portal system are bloodborne to the muscles via the general circulation. They develop to oval infective cysticerci in 60–75 days. After humans ingest inadequately cooked beef, cysticerci attach and grow to sexually mature tapeworms in about 3 mo. Gravid, actively crawling segments are detached from the strobilus in the intestines of infected humans, and these egg-containing segments are passed in the feces. For this reason, individual eggs are difficult to find by fecal flotation procedures. The number of eggs available for cattle

infection may be great, since an infected person often expels eight or nine segments daily, each of which contains 80,000–100,000 eggs. Eggs do not survive desiccation well but retain infectivity in moist pastures for 60–70 days at 20°C (68°F) and 80 days at 10°C (50°F). (See Fig. 2.3.)

   2) *Taenia solium.* The life history of that of *T. solium* is essentially similar to *T. saginata* except that cysticerci occur in humans and swine. The disease produced by *T. solium* in humans therefore, is much more severe than that produced by *T. saginata* and has the added problem of autoinfection. Humans are infected by pork that is improperly cooked or by the ingestion of eggs via the fecal-oral route. Massive infections are usual in swine, and cysticerci show little predilection for specific muscle sites. In light infections, greater numbers are found in muscles of the upper portions of the limbs, abdomen, and diaphragm. The term *Cysticercus cellulosae* is sometimes used to refer to the larval stage in pork measles. (See Fig. 2.4.)

b) *Trichinella spiralis.* *T. spiralis* is a common nematode parasite of carnivorous and omnivorous animals. Pigs, rats, bears, and humans are major hosts. Adults occur in the small intestine, and larval stages occur in musculature. Trichinosis is common in the temperate northern hemisphere and arctic but is less prevalent in the tropics and southern hemisphere.

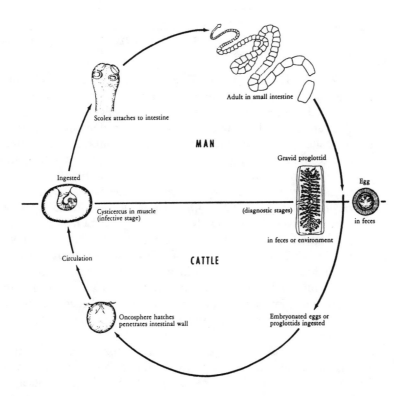

Fig. 2.3. Life cycle of *Taenia saginata*. (Melvin et al. 1959)

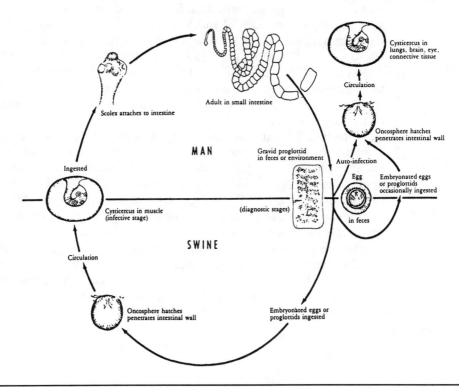

MAN

Adult in small intestine

Scolex attaches to intestine

Ingested

Cysticercus in muscle
(infective stage)

SWINE

Circulation

Oncosphere hatches
penetrates intestinal wall

Gravid proglottid
in feces or environment

(diagnostic stages)

Embryonated eggs or
proglottids ingested

Cysticercus in
lungs, brain, eye,
connective tissue

Circulation

Oncosphere hatches
penetrates intestinal wall

Auto-infection

Egg

in feces

Embryonated eggs
or proglottids
occasionally ingested

Fig. 2.4. Life cycle of *Taenia solium*. (Melvin et al. 1959)

1) *Life cycle.* Transmission of *T. spiralis* from host to host is primarily by ingestion of muscle containing encysted larvae. After ingestion of infected muscle, larvae are released, develop to maturity in the duodenum and jejunum, copulate, and produce new larvae, which are deposited in lacteals and lymph spaces beginning 5 days after infection and continuing for about 40 days. Larvae migrate via lymphatics to the general circulation and to striated muscles. Larvae encyst and must be ingested by a new host for the cycle to continue. (See Fig. 2.5.)

2) *Human infection.* Most *T. spiralis* infections in humans are subclinical. Recent surveys have estimated the prevalence of infection in the general population to be about 2–4 percent, considerably less than the 15–20 percent of 25 yr ago. The case-fatality rate ranges from 1 to 2 percent. Even a few larvae (1–50/g) in human muscle are considered a heavy infection, and 1000/g are considered critical. Clinical infections in domestic animals occur but are not diagnosed except at necropsy. The most common sources of human illness are pork and bear meat. (Table 2.6.)

c) *Toxoplasmosis. Toxoplasma gondii* is a protozoan parasite that can be transmitted to humans through accidental consumption of feces of cats or through ingestion of undercooked meat from infected food animals. The cysts of *T. gondii* will remain viable in the tissues of the infected host for a

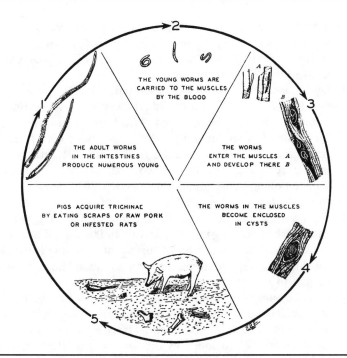

Fig. 2.5. Life cycle of *Trichinella spiralis.* (USDA Yearbook 1942)

Table 2.6. Trichinosis cases by source of infection, United States, 1986

Food		Cases	Percent
Pork		26	60.5
Wild boar	14		
Sausage	7		
Chops	1		
Other	4		
Bear		14	32.6
Cougar		1	2.3
Ground beef		1	2.3
Other		1	2.3
Total		43	100

period of years.

Human disease can range from inapparent subclinical infection to debilitating systemic involvement producing central nervous system damage, chorioretinitis, and abortion. Surveys have revealed that certain individuals (farmers, veterinarians, etc.) have a higher frequency of serologic titers to *T. gondii* than the general population indicating that infection is, to a large degree, an occupational hazard.

Prevention consists of educating the general public, especially women of childbearing age, regarding appropriate hygiene when handling cat feces and ensuring that meat is not consumed raw or poorly cooked.

d) *Endogenous diseases of fish.* Several infectious diseases have been reported in humans for which fish have been a reservoir. Three parasitic disease agents are included in this group.

1) *Diphyllobothrium latum.* The broad tapeworm *D. latum* has intermediate development in freshwater fish; however, some marine species (e.g. salmon) may also be infected. Walleyes and northern pike are two freshwater fish frequently involved. Infections with this tapeworm can result from the preparation of gefilte fish if the mixture is tasted for proper seasoning before it is cooked, or the consumption of sushi. Undercooking is the primary means by which humans become infected with *D. latum.* (See Fig. 2.6.)

2) *Dioctophyma renale.* Humans may become infected with *D. renale* by eating fish containing infective larvae. In the United States, bullhead fish are the important reservoir of this agent. The dog is the definitive host for this parasite, and humans are an accidental host. Transmission from human to human has not been demonstrated.

3) *Anisakis marina.* Another nematode that occurs in marine fish is *A. marina.* This parasite causes severe eosinophilic granulomas or ulceration in the human gastrointestinal tract following ingestion of encapsulated larvae (2 cm long) in the viscera and flesh of raw, salted, or pickled herring, cod, mackerel, or other fish. Marine mammals (dolphins, porpoises, seals) serve as the normal definitive host for the adult stage of *Anisakis.* Larvae are killed by deep freezing ($-20°C/4°F$ for 24 hr). Infections occur mainly in the western states where marine fish occupy the same environment as marine mammals. The current popularity of raw fish (sushi) has increased the number of reported cases.

C. NONMICROBIAL FOOD POISONING

Objectives

1. Describe mechanism of food-associated allergic reactions.
2. Describe how some of the more common chemical intoxicants enter or become part of the food chain, resulting in foodborne disease.
3. Identify and describe sources of food poisoning associated with consumption of inherently poisonous animals.

Text

1. **Naturally Allergenic Foods.** Many foods are naturally allergenic for certain people. Proteins are the substances that usually initiate hypersensitivity reactions. Repeated exposure often results in more serious reactions, varying from a mild pruritic rash to severe abdominal cramps and even death. Clinical signs and symptoms result from histamine release. Although milk and seafood have many documented cases of allergy, meat and poultry are not known to produce allergy.

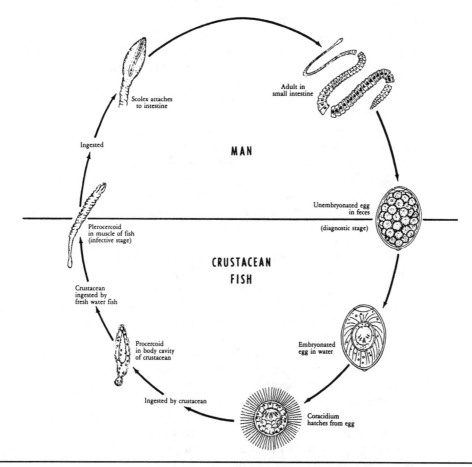

Fig. 2.6. Life cycle of *Diphyllobothrium latum*. (Melvin et al. 1959)

2. **Foodborne Chemicals**. Many chemicals may be transmitted through food.

a) *Nitrate salts*. Preservatives such as nitrates have been used commonly in foods to increase shelf life. Miscalculations and mistaken identity are the usual reasons for overdoses added during processing. The use of nitrate salts is controversial because they may, through a series of reactions, result in the production of nitrosamines that are carcinogenic precursors. The carcinogenic potential of any preservative must be considered before it is used in food.

b) *Sodium nicotinate and sodium sulfite*. Nicotinic acid, or its salts such as sodium nicotinate, has been used to maintain the bright red color in meat by its reaction with hemoglobin and myoglobin. If consumed in quantities of 50 mg or more, it can cause generalized vasodilatation, with cutaneous symptoms of itching, burning, heat, and redness.

Sodium sulfite has been used to mask deterioration in meat. It can be very dangerous if consumed by persons who are allergic to it.

c) *Plant sprays (pesticides)*. Chemicals in the form of insecticides, rodenticides, or herbicides, although not intentionally put on foods, are potential foodborne disease agents. Public education about the dangers of these pesticides is the best way to reduce risk of disease from them. All fruits and vegetables should be assumed to be treated and not safe unless properly handled (washed, peeled, etc). Frequently, the portion of the chemical that is hazardous is a heavy metal, such as in the mercurial and arsenical insecticide sprays used on fruit trees.

d) *Zinc, cadmium, and copper.* Metals may contaminate a food source by a leaching process between the food and its container. Old refrigerator shelves made of cadmium have been used as barbecue grills. Acids from meat cause the cadmium to leach and adhere to the meat, on which it is subsequently ingested. Similarly, galvanized garbage cans may be sources of zinc when used to store fruit drinks at large gatherings. Zinc and cadmium may cause severe abdominal pain and diarrhea. Acidic fruit drinks in copper tubing also may be a source of copper toxicity.

e) *Mercury.* Heavy-metal buildup in animals is an important example of disease agents being transmitted through the food chain. Mercury from a fungicide may enter a watershed and find its way to a commercial fishing bed. Often, the mercury is taken up by microflora that serve as food for more complex organisms in a chain leading to fish and humans (e.g., Minamata disease). Similar intoxications may occur when animals fed chemically treated feeds are eaten by humans (e.g., organic mercury poisoning from eating pork from swine fed treated seed corn). Effluent from an industrial procedure has caused mercury poisoning in humans as a result of drinking-water contamination. Similar signs occur in swine and humans associated with demyelination of the central nervous system.

f) *Drugs.* Foodborne exposure to chemicals may be induced iatrogenically by the veterinarian. The food-animal practitioner must be aware of the potential production of foodborne residues that can result from using drugs such as growth hormones, antibiotics, and insecticides.

g) *Plants.* Animals may concentrate toxic substances in their tissues or milk from ingested plants. When the tissues or milk are eaten by other animals, foodborne disease occurs. White snakeroot is an example of this phenomenon; cattle eat the plants and concentrate the toxic principle in the milk, and it is then consumed by humans. The clinical illness, referred to as *milk sickness* or *tremetol poisoning*, has a geographic distribution associated with the range of these plants.

3. **Poisons from Animals.** Certain animals are inherently poisonous when consumed.
    a) *Toad poisoning.* Toad poisoning is a serious problem when dogs ingest toads (*Bufo* spp.). Clinical signs include paralysis, convulsions, and cardiopulmonary malfunction.
    b) *Scombrotoxin.* This toxin is actually histamine-produced by the action of certain bacteria on histidine present in the muscle of fish. The toxicity of the histamine is potentiated by the presence of co-factors such as cadaverine and putrescine. Certain members of the *Scombridae* family (tuna, bonito, and mackerel) as well as some other dark meat, non-scombroid fish (mahi mahi, herring, bluefish, and amberjack) contain high levels of histidine. Normal fish flesh has approximately 1 mg of histamine/100 gm; concentrations of 20

mg/gm have produced toxicity. The FDA has established 50 mg/100 gm in tuna as a hazardous concentration.

Clinical signs of poisoning include nausea, vomiting, facial flushing, headache, gastric pain, labial edema, urticaria, and an oral burning sensation.

Since affected fish appear normal and the toxin is heat-stable, prevention depends on immediate refrigeration after catching to inhibit bacterial action.

c) *Ciquatoxin*. Evidence indicates that the cause of ciquatera poisoning may be a dinoflagellate associated with reefs. Not all fish of the same species, caught in the same place, at the same time, are toxic. Prevention is difficult because affected fish appear normal. An enzyme immunoassay may prove effective as a screening tool.

The heat-stable toxin produces gastroenteritis, cardiovascular disorders, and neurologic signs, which may persist for months or even years.

d) *Tetrodotoxin*. This toxin is found primarily in pufferfish (hence its common name, pufferfish poisoning) but also may be present in the octopus. Pufferfish species local to the U.S. are not poisonous although, illness has occurred when pufferfish mistakenly included in shipments of fish from Japan have been consumed. (The FDA bans importation of pufferfish.) The heat-stable toxin produces clinical signs similar to those seen with paralytic shellfish poisoning.

D. MILK-ASSOCIATED HEALTH PROBLEMS

Objectives

1. Describe the principal microbial causes of disease from milk and milk products.
2. Describe the residue problems associated with antibiotic therapy of cows.
3. Describe milk contamination problems presented by farm-associated chemicals.
4. Describe the health hazards of radionuclides associated with milk.

Text

1. Principal Bacterial Causes of Disease from Milk or Milk Products

The principal bacterial diseases associated with ingestion of milk or milk products are caused by members of fourteen bacterial genera. The reservoir for these bacteria may be milk-producing mammals (either cows or goats), humans, or contamination from environmental reservoirs. In diseases such as brucellosis, salmonellosis, listeriosis, campylobacteriosis, or tuberculosis, milk may be contaminated with the causative bacteria before it leaves the infected udder. Since milk is an excellent medium for replication of bacteria (propagative vehicle), human carriers of pathogenic bacteria (such as Streptococcus spp., which cause scarlet fever and rheumatic fever) are equally serious sources of contamination. Milkborne transmission of the causative agents of anthrax (*Bacillus anthracis*), nocardiosis (*Nocardia asteroides*), and pasteurellosis (*Pasteurella multocida*) is considered a possibility. (See Tables 2.7 and 2.8.)

a) *Infectious agents other than bacteria*. Risk of milkborne human infection by agents other than bacteria is either remote or uncertain. The protozoal cause of toxoplasmosis, *Toxoplasma gondii*, was discovered in colostrum, and milk

Table 2.7. Bacterial diseases associated with milk or milk products

Diseases Caused by Gram-negative Agents	Cow	Goat	Human	Environment
Brucellosis				
Brucella abortus	+			
Brucella melitensis		+		
Campylobacteriosis				
Campylobacter fetus ssp. *jejuni*	+			
Enteric disease				
Enteropathogenic *Escherichia coli*	+	+	+	
Salmonella dublin	+			
Salmonella typhi			+	
Salmonella spp.	+	+	+	
Shigella spp.			+	
Rat-bite fever				
Streptobacillus moniliformis				+ (rat)
Yersiniosis				
Yersinia enterocolitica	+			+ (feces)

Table 2.8. Bacterial diseases associated with milk or milk products

Diseases Caused by Gram-positive Agents	Cow	Goat	Human	Environment
Listeriosis				
Listeria monocytogenes	+	+	+	+
Diphtheria				
Corynebacterium diphtheriae			+	
Staphylococcal food poisoning				
Enterotoxigenic *Staphylococcus aureus*	+	+	+	
Streptococcal infection				
Streptococcus pyogenes			+	
Other Group A *Streptococcus* spp.			+	
Clostridial foodborne disease				
Clostridium botulinum (intoxication)				+ (soil)
Clostridium perfringens (infection)				+ (soil)
Tuberculosis				
Mycobacterium bovis	+	+		
Mycobacterium tuberculosis			+	
Q fever				
Coxiella burnetii	+	+		

has been implicated as a source of infection for humans. The foot-and-mouth disease (FMD) virus may be shed in milk. The tickborne encephalitis virus (a group B arbovirus) is shed in goat milk, and cases resulting from milkborne transmission have occurred in Asia.

b) *Relative importance of foodborne vs. milk and waterborne transmission.* Although milk is a potentially significant vehicle for transmission of infection to humans, its importance has been reduced drastically in the United States by careful sanitation and the use of pasteurization. Today, disease outbreaks of microbial origin are associated more often with raw milk or inadequately pasteurized (as with recent listeriosis episodes) or manufactured dairy products (particularly botulism from cheese and staphylococcal food poisoning from nonfat dried milk). (See Fig. 2.7.)

2. **Antibiotics.** Whenever a lactating cow is treated by any route with an antibiotic, measurable levels of the antibiotic usually are shed in the milk, even a few days after the last treatment. Antibiotics present in milk are of economic importance because they affect the microorganisms used to ripen cultured dairy products. Persons with hypersensitivity to antibiotics, particularly penicillin, may develop severe allergic reactions if they consume contaminated milk. Penicillin is not

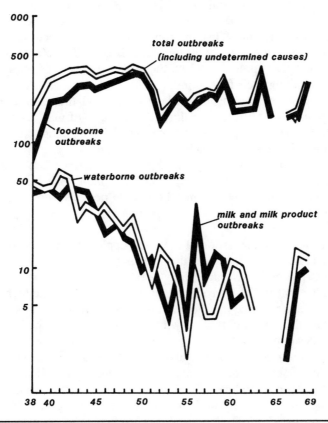

Fig. 2.7. The relative importance of foodborne vs. milk- and waterborne disease outbreaks in the United States, 1938–1968.

inactivated by pasteurization or drying, and levels as low as 0.03 IU/ml have caused severe skin rashes. Of great concern at present is the development of antibiotic-resistant strains of disease-producing microorganisms as a result of the use of antibiotics in food animals. Legally, milk offered for sale must be obtained from healthy cows and must not contain unwholesome substances. A cow treated with antibiotics cannot be considered as healthy, and the presence of antibiotics in the milk constitutes adulteration. Therefore, the milk must be withheld from sale for a specific period of time after therapy (usually 72–96 hr) to ensure that no residues of the therapeutic agent persist. Few drugs are authorized by FDA for use in lactating cows.

3. **Chemicals.** Milk may be contaminated with *toxic chemicals* either before or after it is removed from the cow.

    a) *Insecticides.* Insecticides, particularly chlorinated hydrocarbons, may be absorbed after direct application or from ingestion of foodstuffs treated in the field. As much as 20 percent of an ingested chlorinated hydrocarbon may be excreted in milk. Organic phosphates, however, usually are not excreted in milk. Indiscriminate use of insecticides on farms where milk is handled, or in processing plants, may be a source of contamination. From 25 to 62 percent of market milk supplies sampled during the 1950s contained significant levels of DDT. Since chlorinated hydrocarbons adhere to milk fat, butter contains a much higher proportion of these insecticides. The tolerance level for insecticides in milk products is *zero*. Therefore, these chemicals must not be applied to lactating cows and must be prevented from contaminating their food supply.

    b) *Other drugs excreted in milk.* Many plants and therapeutic agents contain compounds that affect the color, odor, or taste of milk, as well as its safety. Milk from cows fed phenothiazine will develop a pinkish color in a few hours after milking. Cattle that have consumed either white snakeroot (*Eupatorium rugosum*) or jimmyweed (*Haplopappus heterophyllus*) may develop a neurologic disease (trembles) from the plant toxin tremetol. Tremetol poisoning or milk sickness may be fatal in persons who consume milk from affected cows.

4. **Radionuclides.** Contamination of the milk supply with *radionuclides* has become a concern of health officials since the nuclear age. Strontium-90 (radiostrontium), with a half-life of 28 yr, particularly seeks growing bone; iodine-131 (radioiodine), with a half-life of 8 days, concentrates primarily in the thyroid. These two radionuclides are of major concern in milk, and others such as cesium-137 and barium-140 also may find their way into the milk supply. The biologic effects of radionuclides depend on the tissue localization and the type of radiation (alpha, beta, or gamma). Radionuclides may present a health hazard through the milk supply whenever they contaminate the environment in which milk animals are kept or their feed is produced. Significant environmental contamination occurred in several countries as a result of atmospheric testing of nuclear devices. In England, an area of 200–300 sq mi was contaminated with iodine-131 from a reactor fire. Because of this, approximately 250,000 gal milk from 600 exposed herds was condemned. If a contaminating radionuclide has a short half-life (such

as I-131), it is possible to store the contaminated product until the radioactivity decreases to an acceptable level. Decontamination by methods such as ion exchange also is possible.

E. BIBLIOGRAPHY

1. Sources of Food Contamination

Graham, H. D. (ed.). 1980. *The Safety of Foods*. 2d ed. Westport, Conn.: AVI Publishing.
Graham-Rack, B., and R. Binsted. 1973. *Hygiene in Food Manufacturing and Handling*. 2d ed. London: Food Trades Press.
Guthrie, R. R. (ed.). 1988. *Food Sanitation*. 3d ed. New York: Van Nostrand Reinhold.
Libby, J. A. (ed.). 1975. *Meat Hygiene*. 4th ed. Philadelphia: Lea & Febiger.

2. Microbial Causes of Foodborne Disease

Arnon, S. S. 1980. Review of present knowledge about a newly recognized form of botulism in which honey has been implicated. *Annu. Rev. Med.* 31:541-60.
Arnon, S. S., K. Damus, and J. Chin. 1981. Infant botulism: Epidemiology and relation to sudden death syndrome. *Epidemiol. Rev.* 3:45-66.
Arnon, S. S., K. Damus, B. Thompson, T. F. Midura, and J. Chin. 1982. Protective role of human milk against sudden death from infant botulism. *J. Pediatr.* 100(4):568-73.
Beaver, P. C., and R. C. Jung. 1985. *Animal Agents and Vectors of Human Disease*. 5th ed. Philadelphia: Lea & Febiger.
Benenson, A. S. (ed.). 1985. *Control of Communicable Diseases in Man*. 14th ed. Washington, D.C.: American Public Health Association.
Blaser, M. J., D. N. Taylor, and R. A. Feldman. 1983. Epidemiology of *Campylobacter jejuni* infections. Epidemiol. Rev. 5:157-76.
Bryan, F. L. 1972. Emerging foodborne diseases. I. Their surveillance and epidemiology. II. Factors that contribute to outbreaks and their control. *J. Milk Food Technol.* 35:618-25, 632-38.
Chichester, C. O., and H. D. Graham (eds.). 1975. *Microbial Safety of Fishery Products*. New York: Academic Press.
Cox, L. 1983. Interstate common-source outbreak of staphylococcal food poisoning: North Carolina, Pennsylvania. *MMWR* 32(14):183-89.
Dirks, T. 1982. A foodborne outbreak of streptoccal pharyngitis: Portland, Oregon. *MMWR* 31(1-2):3-5.
Doughty, S. C. 1984. Foodborne botulism. *MMWR* 33(2):22-23.
Genigeorgis, C. A. 1981. Factors affecting the probability of growth of pathogenic microorganisms in foods. *J. Am. Vet. Med. Assoc.* 179(12):1410-17.
Gill, O. N., W. D. Cubitt, D. A. McSwiggan, B. M. Watney, and C. L. Bartlett. 1983. Illness associated with fish and shellfish in England and Wales. *Br. Med. J.* 287 (6401):1284-85.
Hobbs, B.C. and J. H. B. Christian (eds.). 1973. *Microbiological Safety of Foods*. London: Academic Press.
Holmberg, S. D., and P. A. Blake. 1984. Staphylococcal food poisoning in the United States: New facts and old misconceptions. *J. Am. Med. Assoc.* 251(4):487-89.
Hopkins, R. S., R. Olmsted, and G. R. Istre. 1984. Endemic *Campylobacter jejuni* infection in Colorado: Identified risk factors. *Am. J. Public Health* 74(3):249-50.
Hughes, J. M., and C. O. Tacket. 1983. Sausage poisoning revisited. *Arch. Intern. Med.* 143(3):425.
Kotula, A. W., and N. O. Stern. 1984. The importance of *Campylobacter jejuni* to the meat industry: A review. *J. Sci.* 58(6): 1561-66.

Kreuzer, R. (ed.). 1972. *Fish Inspection and Quality Control*. London: Fishing News (Books).

Lewis, K. H., and K. Cassel, Jr. (eds.). 1964. *Botulism: Proceeding of a Symposium*. USPHS Publ. No. 999-FP-1. Washington, D.C.: U.S. Government Printing Office.

Libby, J. A. (ed.). 1975. *Meat Hygiene*. 4th ed. Philadelphia: Lea & Feiber.

Marks, M. I. 1980. *Yersinia enterocolitica* gastroenteritis: A prospective study of clinical, bacteriologic and epidemiologic features. *J. Pediatr.* 96(1):26-31.

Melconian, A. K., Y. Brun, and J. Fleurette. 1983. Enterotoxin production, phage typing and serotyping of *Staphylococcus aureus* strains isolated from clinical materials. *J. Hyg.* 91 (2):235-42.

Melvin, D. M., M. M. Brooke, and E. H. Sadun. 1959. *Life Charts: Common Intestinal Helminths of Man*. Atlanta, Ga.: Communicable Disease Center.

Miller, D. P., and E. D. Everett. 1983. Bacterial enteritis. *Mo. Med.* 80(5):241-48.

Morris, J. G., J. D. Snyder, R. Wilson, and R. A. Feldman. 1983. Infant botulism in the United States: An epidemiologic study of cases occurring outside of California. *Am. J. Public Health* 73(12):1385-88.

Mossel, D. A. A. 1982. *Microbiology of Foods*. 3d ed. The University of Utrecht, Faculty of Veterinary Medicine.

Norkrans, G., and A. Svedhem. 1982. Epidemiological aspects of *Campylobacter jejuni* enteritis. *J. Hyg.* 89(1):163-70.

Pether, J. Y., and E. O. Caul. 1983. An outbreak of foodborne gastroenteritis in two hospitals associated with a Norwalk-like virus. *J. Hyg.* 91(2):343-50.

Prescott, J. F., and D. L. Munroe. 1982. *Campylobacter jejuni* enteritis in man and domestic animals. *J. Am. Vet. Med. Assoc.* 181(12):1524-30.

Ray, K., P. Aggarval, and A. M. Rai Chowdhuri. 1983. Simultaneous isolation of *Salmonella stanley* and *S. oranienburg* from an outbreak of food poisoning. *Indian J. Med. Res.* 77:602-4.

Reimann, H., and F. L. Bryan (eds.). 1979. *Food-borne Infections and Intoxications*. 2d ed. New York: Academic Press.

Rodricks, J. V., C. W. Helleltine, and M. A. Mehlman (eds.). 1977. *Mycotoxins in Human and Animal Health*. Park Forest South, Ill.: Pathotox Publishers.

Roueche, B. 1953. *Eleven Blue Men*. New York: Berkley Publishing.

Sellin, L. C. 1984. Botulism: An update. *Milit. Med.* 149(1):12-16.

Shandera, W. X., C. O. Tacket, and F. A. Blake. 1983. Food poisoning due to *Clostridium perfringens* in the United States. *J. Infect. Dis.* 147(1):167-70.

Shane, S. M., and M. S. Montrose. 1985. The occurrence and significance of *Camplyobacter jejuni* in man and animals. *Vet. Res. Commun.* 9:167-98.

United Nations. World Health Organization. 1974. *Food-borne Disease: Methods of Sampling and Examination in Surveillance Programs. Report of a WHO Study Group*. WHO Tech. Rep. Ser. No. 543. Geneva: World Health Organization.

_____. 1974. *Fish and Shellfish Hygiene*. WHO Tech. Rep. Ser. No. 550. Geneva: World Health Organization.

U.S. Army Medical Service. 1962. *Inspection of Waterfoods*. Washington, D.C.: U.S. Government Printing Office.

U.S. Department of Health, Education, and Welfare. Public Health Service, Center for Disease Control. 1978. *Brucellosis Surveillance*. Washington, D.C.: U.S. Government Printing Office.

_____. 1982. *Salmonella Surveillance*. Washington, D.C.: U.S. Government Printing Office.

_____. 1983. *Foodborne and Waterborne Disease Outbreaks*. Washington, D.C.: U.S. Government Printing Office.

U.S. Department of Health and Human Services. Public Health Service. Centers for Disease Control. 1988. *Water-Related Disease Outbreaks, 1985*. Washington, D.C.:

U.S. Government Printing Office.

_____. 1988. *Salmonella Isolates from Humans in the United States, 1984-1986.* Washington, D.C.: U.S. Government Printing Office.

Wilson, R., J. G. Morris, V. D. Snyder, and R. A. Feldman. 1982. Clinical characteristics of infant botulism in the United States: A study of the non-California cases. *Pediatr. Infect. Dis.* 1(3):148-50.

3. Nonmicrobial Food Poisoning

Bond, E. J. (ed.). *Manual of Fumigation for Insect Control.* 3d ed. New York: Unipub.

Brown, A. W. A. 1978. *Ecology of Pesticides.* New York: John Wiley & Sons.

Brown, M. A., J. V. Thom, G. L. Orth, P. Cova, and J. Juarez. 1964. Food poisoning involving zinc contamination. *Arch. Environ. Health.* 8: 657-60.

Buck, W. B., G. D. Osweiler, and G. A. Van Gelder. 1984. *Clinical and Diagnostic Veterinary Toxicology.* 2d ed. Dubuque, Iowa: Kendall-Hunt.

Catsimpoolas, N. (ed.). 1977. *Immunological Aspects of Foods.* Westport, Conn.: AVI Publishing.

Curley, A., V. A. Sedlak, E. F. Girling, et al. 1971. Organic mercury identified as the cause of poisoning in humans and hogs. *Science* 172:65-67.

Dickinson, G. 1982. Scombroid fish poisoning syndrome. *Ann. Emerg. Med.* 11(9):487-89.

Fairchild, E. J. (ed.). 1978. *Agricultural Chemicals and Pesticides.* Fort Lee, N.J.: Jack K. Burgess, Inc.

Hayes, W. J., Jr. 1975. *Toxicology of Pesticides.* Baltimore: Williams & Wilkins.

Humphreys, D. J. 1988. *Veterinary Toxicology.* 3d ed. Philadelphia: Saunders.

Ivie, G. W., and H. W. Dorough (eds.). 1977. *Fate of Pesticides in Large Animals.* New York: Academic Press.

Kingsbury, J. M. 1964. *Poisonous Plants of the United States and Canada.* Englewood Cliffs, N.J.: Prentice-Hall.

Kumpulainen, J., and P. Koivistoinen. 1977. Fluorine in foods. Residue Rev. 68:37-57.

Lapham, S., R. Vanderly, R. Brackbill, and M. Tikkauen. 1983. Illness associated with elevated levels of zinc in fruit punch: New Mexico. MMWR 32(19):257-58.

Leonard, B. J. (ed.). 1978. *Toxicological Aspects of Food Safety.* New York: Springer-Verlag.

Lucas, J. 1974. *Our Polluted Food: A Survey of the Risks.* New York: John Wiley & Sons.

Nelson, N., chairman. 1975. *Principles for Evaluating Chemicals in the Environment.* Washington, D.C.: National Academy of Sciences.

Poskanzer, D. C., and A. L. Herbst. 1977. Epidemiology of vaginal adenosis and adenocarcinoma associated with exposure to stilbestrol in utero. *Cancer* 39:1892-95.

Press, E. and L. Yeager. 1962. Food "poisoning" due to sodium nicotinate. *Am. J. Pub. Health.* 52:1720-28.

Radeleff, R. D. 1970. *Veterinary Toxicology.* 2d ed. Philadelphia: Lea & Febiger.

United Nations. World Health Organization. 1971. *Evaluation of Some Pesticide Residues in Food.* WHO Pestic. Residues Ser. No. 1. Geneva: World Health Organization.

_____. 1972. *Evaluation of Mercury, Lead, Cadmium and the Food Additives Amaranth, Diethylpyrocarbonate, and Octyl Gallate.* WHO Food Addit. Ser. No. 4. Geneva: World Health Organization.

_____. 1972. *A Review of the Technological Efficacy of Some Antioxidants and Synergists.* WHO Food Addit. Ser. No. 3. Geneva: World Health Organization.

4. Milk-associated Health Problems

Anderson, P. H. R., and D. M. Stone. 1955. Staphylococcal food poisoning associated with spray-dried milk. *J. Hyg.* (*Camb.*) 53:387-97.

Bahna, S. L. 1978. Control of milk allergy: A challenge for physicians, mothers and industry. *Ann. Allergy* 41:1-12.

Beware of the cow. 1974. *Lancet* 2(787):30-31.

Black, R. E., R. J. Jackson, T. Tsai, M. Medvesky, M. Shayegani, J. C. Feeley, K. I. E. MacLeod, and A. M. Wakelee. 1978. Epidemic *Yersinia enterocolitica* infection due to contaminated chocolate milk. *N. Engl. J. Med.* 298:76-79.

Fries, G. F. 1978. Distribution and kinetics of polybrominated biphenyls and selected chlorinated hydrocarbons in farm animals. *J. Am. Vet. Med. Assoc.* 173:1479-84.

Garza, C., and N. S. Scrimshaw. 1976. Relationship of lactose intolerance to milk intolerance in young children. *Am. J. Clin. Nutr.* 29:1902-6.

Graivier, L., N. E. Harper, and G. Currarino. 1977. Milk-curd bowel obstruction in the newborn infant. *J. Am. Med. Assoc.* 238:1050-52.

Henry, E. T. 1979. Pasteurization for safe milk. *J. Am. Vet. Med. Assoc.* 175:1138, 1154 (letter).

Hird, D. W. 1979. Hazards of certified raw milk. *J. Am. Vet. Med. Assoc.* 175:874-75 (letter).

James, L. F., and W. J. Hartley. 1977. Effects of milk from animals fed locoweed on kittens, calves, and lambs. *Am. J. Vet. Res.* 38:1263-65.

Johnson, A. E. 1976. Changes in calves and rats consuming milk from cows fed chronic lethal doses of *Senecio jacobaea* (tansy rag-wort). *Am J. Vet. Res.* 37:107-10.

Lamm, S. H., and J. F. Rosen. 1974. Lead contamination in milks fed to infants: 1972-1973. *Pediatrics* 53:137-41, 142-46.

Larson, B. L., and K. E. Ebner. 1960. Strontium-90 and milk, considerations on SR-90 and the role of milk in our diet. *J. Dairy Sci.* 43:119-24.

Marth, E. H., and B. E. Ellickson. 1959. Problems created by the presence of antibiotics in milk and milk products. *J. Milk Food Technol.* 22:266-72.

Matthysse, J. G. 1974. Insecticides used on dairy cattle and in dairy barns: Toxicity to man and cattle, hazards to the consumer and the environment. *J. Milk Food Technol.* 37:255-64.

Milk-borne outbreaks of *Salmonella typhimurium*. 1977. *Br. Med. J.* 1(6076):1606.

Mol, H. 1975. *Antibiotics and Milk*. Rotterdam: A. A. Balkema.

Myers, J. A., and J. H. Steele. 1969. *Bovine Tuberculosis in Man and Animals*. St. Louis: Green.

Pamukcu, A. M., E. Erturk, S. Yalciner, U. Milli, and G. T. Bryan. 1978. Carcinogenic and mutagenic activities of milk from cows fed bracken fern (*Pteridium aquilinum*). *Cancer Res.* 38:1556-60.

Richardson, G. H., (ed.). 1985. *Standard Methods for the Examination of Dairy Products*. 15th ed. Washington, D.C.: American Public Health Association.

Riemann, H. P., M. E. Meyer, J. H. Theis, G. Kelso, and D. E. Behymer. 1975. Toxoplasmosis in an infant fed unpasteurized goat milk. *J. Pediatr.* 87:573-76.

Schiemann, D. A., and S. Toma. 1978. Isolation of *Yersinia enterocolitica* from raw milk. *Appl. Environ. Microbiol.* 35:54-58.

Small, R. G., and J. C. M. Sharp. 1979. A milk-borne outbreak due to *Salmonella dublin*. *J. Hyg. (Camb.)* 82:95-100.

Spink, W. W. 1956. *The Nature of Brucellosis*. Minneapolis: University of Minnesota Press.

Stone, W., and F. W. Smith. 1973. Infection of mammalian hosts by milk-borne nematode larvae: A review. *Exp. Parasitol.* 34:306-13.

Svabic-Vlahovic, M., D. Pantic, M. Pavicic, and J. H. Bryner. 1988. Transmission of *Listeria monocytogenes* from mother's milk to her baby and to puppies. *Lancet* 2(8621):1201.

Tacket, C. O., J. P. Narain, R. Sattin, J. P. Lofgren, C. Konigsberg, R. C. Rendtorff, A. Rausa, B. R. Davis, and M. L. Cohen. 1984. A multistate outbreak of infections caused by *Yersinia enterocolitica* transmitted by pasteurized milk. *J. Am. Med. Assoc.*

251(4):483-86.

Taylor, P. R., W. M. Wernstein, and J. H. Bryner. 1979. *Camplyobacter fetus* infection in humans: Association with raw milk. *Am. J. Med.* 66:779-83.

Woodruff, C. W. 1976. Milk intolerances. *Nutr. Rev.* 34:33-37.

3 Consumer Protection

A. PREVENTING FOODBORNE DISEASE

Objectives

1. Describe the practical aspects involved in applying the following three principles of foodborne disease prevention:
   a) Prevent contamination.
   b) Inhibit pathogen growth.
   c) Kill pathogens.
2. Describe the problems of unacceptable drug and chemical residues in meat and milk, including control methods used.
3. Describe the hazard analysis critical control point technique for ensuring that foods of animal origin are safe for human consumption.

Text

1. **Factors in Preventing Foodborne Disease.** Several factors are essential for foodborne bacterial disease to occur. They are (1) pathogenic bacteria present, (2) a source of contamination (e.g., knife, cutting board, hands, mouth), (3) a medium in which the bacteria can grow, (4) proper environmental relationships (e.g., time, temperature, moisture), and (5) consumption of a sufficient quantity. Four food-processing fundamentals essential to preventing foodborne disease are (1) *preventing contamination* of foods during each step of processing, especially when handling foods already cooked, (2) *inhibiting growth* of organisms in foods already contaminated, (3) *inactivating pathogens* to prevent foodborne disease, and (4) *controlling residues*.

2. **Preventing Microbial Contamination**
   a) *Personal hygiene*. Contamination of food can be prevented or at least minimized by practicing good personal hygiene at all points along the food

chain.

b) *Equipment*. Preventing contamination of food products includes using properly cleaned equipment. A three-step process, involving washing with cleaning compounds and water, rinsing, and sanitizing effectively, cleans utensils and equipment. The rinsing procedure removes excess cleaning compounds. Sanitizing may be done by immersion in hot water (76.7°C/ 170°F) for at least 30 sec or by using a chemical rinse. Three factors are important in the chemical method: (1) immersion time, (2) solution or water temperature, and (3) concentration of active ingredients. These factors vary depending on the chemical used.

Spread of microorganisms from contaminated food to other foods can be prevented if separate utensils are used for each. If the same equipment must be used, it should be cleaned thoroughly and disinfected between uses. Of prime consideration is cross-contamination between raw and cooked foods.

c) *Ingredients*. Unwholesome ingredients can contaminate a prepared food product. Only inspected foods with undamaged containers should be used.

3. **Inhibiting Growth of Microorganisms.** Foods may be divided into three categories based on their ability to support bacterial growth: (1) those that *readily support growth* (propagative vehicles), (2) those that will *permit survival* but not multiplication, and (3) those that actually kill pathogens.

Microorganisms have specific needs for growth and multiplication. By restricting certain factors in the organisms' environment, growth can be inhibited or at least retarded. Factors that can be manipulated are food (e.g., by preservatives), moisture, temperature, pH, and time.

a) *Low temperatures*. Foodborne disease of microbial origin is prevented by inhibiting growth of microorganisms in food. Most pathogens are mesophilic organisms and grow best at temperatures between 4.4°C (40°F) and 60°C (140°F). Foods should be stored at temperatures outside of this range. If a cooked food is to be cooled, it should be done as rapidly as possible. With large quantities of food, it is difficult both to achieve adequate heat penetration and a rapid cooling time.

After food is chilled, it should be refrigerated at 4.4°C (40°F) or less. Clostridial spores and staphylococcal toxins are not destroyed by normal cooking; thus preventing their introduction and inhibiting their growth is relied on to effectively prevent outbreaks of foodborne disease.

Precooling ingredients helps inhibit microbial growth during preparation. In sausage production, meat processors often add ice instead of water to cool the mixture.

b) *High temperatures*. If hot foods must be held for a period before serving, the temperature should be in excess of 60°C (140°F) at the center.

c) *Moisture*. The amount of water available to microorganisms is expressed as water activity (*Aw* level). Water activity is defined as the ratio of water vapor pressure of the food (p) to that of pure water (po) at the same temperature:

$$Aw = p/po$$

Aw level should not be confused with water content. Two foods of the same water content may have different *Aw* levels. Fresh meat, fish, and milk usually have an *Aw* level of .98 or higher; sausage and cheese will be between .85 and .93. Even though microorganisms may survive for some period of time at unfavorable *Aw* levels, knowledge of optimum *Aw* levels is useful in determining potential hazards. Salmonellae and *Escherichia coli*, for example, have an optimum *Aw* level of .95, whereas *Staphylococcus aureus* has an optimum level of .86.

d) *Time*. Although food should be consumed immediately after preparation, this is not always practical. If all conditions are favorable, bacterial growth is cumulative and includes lag and logarithmic phases. Generally, foods held between 4.4°C (40°F) and 60°C (140°F) should be eaten within 4 hr. Some variability exists because inoculum size may vary.

4. **Destroying Pathogens.** Vegetative forms of microorganisms are killed by thorough cooking, whereas spores and some toxins usually are not destroyed. Because complete and adequate heat penetration is more difficult when large quantities of food are cooked, food should be cooked in small quantities when possible.

5. **Controlling Chemical Adulteration.** The industrial revolution had far-reaching effects, among them a dramatic change in techniques for producing food, particularly those of animal origin. Technology took the responsibility for the purity of food out of the kitchen and relegated it to the increasingly complex food chain described in Chapter 1.

   Concomitant with these technological advances was an increased potential for the adulteration of foods of animal origin with toxic materials.

a) *Sources of chemical adulteration*. A food is *adulterated* whenever it contains any chemical that may render it injurious to health or otherwise unfit for human food. Meat and poultry may become adulterated with unacceptable concentrations of chemicals during production of the animals before slaughter or during processing, packaging, or storage of the meat after slaughter. During their growth, animals may be intentionally or inadvertently exposed to antibiotics, sulfonamides, growth-promoting substances, mycotoxins, pesticides, toxic metals, and radionuclides. Any of these may persist at slaughter and are considered *residues*. Some chemical may be deliberately added during processing or packaging, either legally or illegally, and these are considered *additives*. Other chemical *contaminants* may occur unintentionally during processing, packaging, or storage, such as those that result from leaching of chemical constituents from the packaging materials.

b) *Standard measures of acceptable concentrations*. Health risks from residues in food are determined in relation to the toxicity or hazard of the chemical and the likelihood of exposure (i.e., consuming it in a given food). Although the toxicity of a chemical in food remains relatively constant, exposure to humans varies greatly among foods of animal origin, depending on the likelihood of exposure of the food animal to the chemical. Average daily intake is another important factor in determining exposure-related risk, especially for milkborne residues and infants inasmuch as milk represents a much-higher-than-average portion of their diet.

   In the United States, the maximum acceptable residue concentrations in foods are established by the Environmental Protection Agency (EPA) for pesticides and by the FDA for animal drugs and unavoidable environmental contaminants. The concentrations, designated in parts per million (ppm) or parts per billion (ppb), are referred to as *tolerances*. International standards, available for use by all countries, have been developed for more than 2000 compounds by the joint FAO/WHO Codex Alimentarius Commission and are referred to as *maximum residue limits* (MRLs).

Inasmuch as most data used to establish these limits are derived from animal studies, an "uncertainty factor" is added beyond the level demonstrated to cause no observable effect for an extra margin of safety. Usually, the uncertainty factor is 100- to 1000-fold for short- and long-term hazards other than cancer. The level for cancer represents a dietary exposure that ensures (at a 95 percent confidence level) that a risk of 1 in a million will not be exceeded during a 40-year lifetime.

c) *Nitrates and nitrites*. These chemicals are additives used in meat and meat products to protect against botulism, to develop cured meat flavor and color, and to retard rancidity during storage. Nitrites are the active salts. Nitrates convert to nitrites over time and continue the desired action.

In recent years the occurrence of nitrosamines, which are produced by the interaction of nitrites and secondary or tertiary amines in meat, has been a subject of concern. Dimethylnitrosamine (DMN), the simplest member of the nitrosamines, is a strong hepatotoxic agent. Of among 130 nitroso compounds tested, more than 80 percent were found to be carcinogenic.

On the other hand, elimination of nitrites may result in an increase in the number of cases of botulism among consumers.

In an effort to retain the positive effects of nitrites but reduce their hazards, the USDA has banned the inclusion of nitrates in seasoning premixes and placed a ceiling of 120 ppm in bacon.

d) *Types of residues*. Livestock and poultry producers are recognizing that they must consider themselves food producers rather than merely livestock or poultry feeders. Two of the major responsibilities of the veterinary profession are to advise food-animal producers how to eliminate financial loss as the result of carcass adulteration resulting from unlawful residues and to protect consumers from exposure to food containing unlawful concentrations of residues. Several types of residue are found in foods of animal origin: industrial chemicals, agricultural chemicals, and veterinary therapeutic agents. The former two categories are of occasional clinical concern to veterinarians, usually manifested as herd problems. The latter, the therapeutic agents, are of constant concern to veterinarians involved in the production of food animals.

e) *Agricultural and industrial chemicals*. Although these chemicals are responsible for only occasional clinical episodes in food animals, they may be more important as causes of adulteration. Therefore, veterinarians need to be aware of how agricultural and industrial chemicals can contaminate animal feed and water sources if they are to alert their food-animal producer clients to these dangers. For example, when heptachlor-treated seed grains were used as feed for dairy cattle, poultry, and swine, extensive losses resulted from condemnation of adulterated meat and milk. Heptachlor persists for long periods in body fat. Polybrominated and polychlorinated biphenyls are industrial chemicals that persist in fat, cause clinical signs in animals, have been noted as residue producers, and have caused problems as a result of feed contamination.

f) *Veterinary therapeutic agents.* A decision regarding therapy of any food animal must first be justified on a cost-benefit basis that takes into consideration the value of the healthy animal, the cost of therapy, and the salvage value of the unhealthy animal (Fig. 3.1).

   1) *Hormones.* Use of diethylstilbestrol (DES) will produce a 1000-lb beef animal 30 days sooner than is required for a nontreated animal and will save about 500 lb of feed. This 10 to 12 percent increase in efficiency could save about 7.7 billion lb of feed annually in the United States.

   Concern about the causal association between sex hormones and neoplasia, however, resulted in the passage in 1958 of the Delaney Amendment to the Food, Drug, and Cosmetic Act prohibiting the use of potential carcinogens. This was modified in 1962 to permit carcinogens to be used in animals if *none* was found in edible portions of the carcass. At that time, the minimum amount detectable was 100 ppm. Anything less than this equaled zero. At the present time, techniques exist for detecting levels as low as a few ppb. During the late 1970s, several actions were taken by FDA to eliminate all use of DES in cattle.

   2) *Antibiotics and sulfonamides.* More than 40 percent of antibacterial agents produced in the United States are for animals. Nearly 100 percent of poultry, 90 percent of swine, and 60 percent of cattle receive antibacterial feed supplements. About 70 percent of United States beef, by carcass weight, has received growth-promoting supplementation. Most often, antibiotic residues appear in meat or meat products because of failure to observe proper withdrawal periods after therapy. This therapy may be in response to clinical disease or may be preventive in nature, such as in dry-cow therapy or feed additives. Utilization of antibiotics in feed to promote growth started in the 1940s and has been continued with very little control until recently. Concern about antibiotic resistance has prompted studies and recommendations, such as the Swann Report

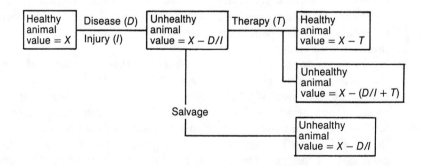

Fig. 3.1. Decision algorithm for food-animal therapy.

from the United Kingdom that urged eliminating or at least severely curtailing use of medicated feeds. In 1970 a special task force was appointed by the FDA to study the use of antibiotics in animal feeds. The group concluded:

(a) Antibiotic and sulfonamide drug use, especially in growth-promotant and subtherapeutic amounts, favors selection and development of single- and multiple-antibiotic-resistant and R-plasmid-bearing bacteria.

(b) Animals receiving subtherapeutic and/or therapeutic amounts of antibiotic and sulfonamide drugs in feeds may serve as a reservoir of antibiotic-resistant pathogens and nonpathogens. These reservoirs of pathogens can produce human infections.

(c) The prevalence of multiresistant, R-plasmid-bearing pathogenic and nonpathogenic bacteria in animals has increased and has been related to use of antibiotics and sulfonamide drugs.

(d) Antibiotic-resistant organisms have been found in meat and meat products.

(e) There has been an increase in prevalence of antibiotic- and sulfonamide-resistant bacteria in humans.

Veterinarians may be held legally responsible for utilizing antibiotics in such a manner that illegal concentrations of medications are found in carcasses of food animals. Veterinarians also may be held responsible for failure to advise clients of potential residue problems. Many producers, for example, do not realize that veal calves can have measurable residue concentrations when nursing dams are treated with antibiotics. Even pooled colostrum fed to calves may produce residues.

3) *Control of therapeutic-agent residues*

(a) *By the practitioner.* Food-animal practitioners must be familiar with the pharmacology of drugs they use for therapy or in preventive medicine programs, in particular, the required withdrawal times. Drugs with a short biologic half-life, such as penicillin, usually create very few residue problems. Those with a longer half-life, such as streptomycin, are more likely to be associated with violative concentrations in meat or milk.

(1) Guidelines concerning drugs approved for use in food animals and appropriate withdrawal times are published by the Center for Veterinary Medicine (CVM) of the FDA. In addition, many veterinary organizations and extension programs provide information regarding prevention of residue problems. Lactating dairy cows present the greatest problem inasmuch as only a handful of drugs are approved for use without some withholding of milk.

(2) Drug manufacturers are required to furnish information about withdrawal times for medications they manufacture and sell. Reading the label and adhering to stated guidelines will avoid potential problems. Drugs such as sulfamethazine persist in the environment, and this factor must be considered as well in preventing residues.

(3) Identification of treated animals and maintenance of a permanent record that documents drugs used, route and date of administration, and recommended withdrawal periods will avoid possible legal judgments against the practitioner. This is especially important when using *extra-label* (unapproved) drug therapy. Extra-label use involves a careful decision by a veterinarian to use a product in a species for which it has not been specifically approved. However, some drugs, such as chloramphenicol, have always been *prohibited* from use in food animals and any administration would be an illegal misuse.

(4) Test kits are available for the veterinarian to use on the farm to detect antibiotic residue concentrations in meat and milk before shipment.

(b) *By regulatory agencies*

(1) *Milk.* In addition to standard tests for butterfat, protein content, and somatic cell count, milk is now routinely examined for the presence of antibiotic residues upon receipt in dairy plants. The tests currently in use utilize inhibition of growth of antibiotic-susceptible organisms, (e.g., *Bacillus subtilis* or *B. stearothermophilus*) that can detect concentrations of penicillin as low as 0.004 IU/ml. A variation of these tests can be used by milk-truck drivers as a screening procedure at the farm.

(2) *Meat.* Detection of antibiotic-adulterated meat depends on two things: the professional expertise of the veterinarian and the USDA national residue program. Veterinarians working in an inspection program must know the antemortem signs associated with exposure to naturally occurring toxicants, drugs, pesticides, feed additives, and environmental contaminants as well as the postmortem lesions produced. They must be familiar with food-animal production practices and be able to anticipate potential problems such as those seen among cull dairy cows and newborn or "bob" veal calves. Finally, they must be able to collect limited case histories to help identify an adulterant and its source.

The USDA currently is capable of testing slaughtered animals for more than 400 drugs, pesticides, herbicides, industrial chemicals, and heavy metals. This detection program consists of two parts, *surveillance* and *monitoring,* which are means of gathering information from a subset (sample) of a population in order to make inferences regarding the population as a whole. Both involve samples that are representative (by means of random selection, etc.) of the population in question. These techniques may involve *testing* (collection of tissue specimens from individuals in a population sample for analysis).

Surveillance is designed to detect components of the livestock and poultry population in which residue problems exist, to determine the extent of the problem, and to evaluate the impact of actions initiated to reduce the problem. The information obtained by surveillance is specifically intended to provide the basis for a decision on which of a range of predetermined actions to take. One possible action would be testing animals presented for slaughter (see below). Surveillance results in rapid awareness among the producers *with* the problem (in the problem population); it has less impact on producers *without* the problem (not in the problem population).

Monitoring also answers questions regarding residues in (nonproblem) populations, using the same techniques as surveillance, but it is not intended to trigger action (control). Combining monitoring and surveillance results provides a picture of the overall population (e.g., beef cows + dairy cows = all cattle).

Testing all the animals or representatives from every lot (rather than merely testing a sample of individuals or lots) presented for slaughter from problem populations with high residue rates further stimulates producer interest in problem solving, as well as providing enhanced consumer protection with greater assurance of detecting adulteration. Testing is one tool to reduce residues in problem populations. It detects animals with violative concentrations of residues and prevents them from entering the food supply. A by-product of such testing is its impact on problem producers. Discretionary testing of individual animals or lots with injection sites or other clinical evidence suggesting a residue problems as well as testing animals from owners with history of residue problems, is a valuable tool in the overall consumer-protection program.

A producer found in violation must have two consecutive lots of animals (at least five animals each) tested and found free from residues before being released from further testing of all animals presented for slaughter. The carcasses are retained until the test is completed. In the past, this could take 5-12 days. Now the Swab Test on Premises (STOP) is used. Muscle, kidney, or liver is swabbed, plated on a *B. subtilis* culture, and incubated for 12 hr at 29°C (84.2°F). If results are positive, specimens are sent to a laboratory for confirmation. Using the STOP program, FSIS can test 10 times the number of animals that were tested previously. A modification of this test, the Live Animal Swab Test (LAST) is used with urine so that producers can screen animals before slaughter.

g) *Preventing violative residues.* To be most effective in advising food animal producer clients, veterinarians should be prepared to develop an efficient program of residue prevention. This involves examining *all* critical points in the client's production enterprise in which residue problems may evolve. Elements to consider include the following:

1) Animals   (source and/or history, identification, individual medications, withdrawal periods)
2) Feed   (source, possible pesticide or other contamination, separation of

medicated from non-medicated, water supply)

3) Management   (trained personnel, records for feed and medication)

4) Environment   (isolation pens; storage of drugs and other chemicals, such as pesticides, including proper labeling; mixers and other feed handling equipment; bioaccumulation by recycling in manure)

5) Quality control   (tests of milk and/or urine, tests of samples of purchased feed if uncertain origin)

6. **Hazards Analysis Critical Control Points (HACCP).** The HACCP technique is an application of a well-established procedure, used in a variety of production systems, to monitor quality. Whether the product is automobiles, cans of beans, or shoes, the approach is essentially the same. The production process is monitored at points that logic and experience have indicated to be potential problems. A good monitoring system begins with the raw materials and continues to the finished product.

The HACCP is a variation of this technique in that the critical points for monitoring are selected on the basis of potential for the introduction of hazards to human health. The emphasis is on such hazards, rather than quality as related to consumer acceptance.

The HACCP technique involves 4 steps:

a) A schematic or flow chart of the entire production, processing, and distribution procedure is developed. For beef, this would begin with production of the raw material on the farm or in the feedlot, progress through the slaughtering plant, and end at the delivery point of the finished product (retail market).

b) Points in the flow chart that are potential trouble spots are identified. The emphasis regarding "trouble" under the HACCP technique is on hazards to human health, not on production efficiency or on esthetics. The selection of these potential trouble spots is based on a thorough knowledge of the hazards involved (physical, chemical, or microbial) and experience with the production system in use. The latter is important because, even though basic procedures are similar, each stage in production, processing, and delivery has different trouble spots as a result of differing physical facilities, equipment, sources of raw material, and personnel.

c) Appropriate surveillance procedures are selected. The procedures depend on the particular hazard of concern. A potential hazard associated with employee activity would best be monitored visually. Records of production and purchase are important in monitoring feed-associated hazards. Organoleptic procedures are appropriate for detecting potential hazards associated with carcasses and finished products. Testing feed ingredients, tissue samples, or environmental surfaces may be essential to detect chemical and microbiologic contamination.

Timing and frequency of surveillance is as important as the point of sampling. Equipment swabs, for instance, may reveal nearly sterile surfaces at 8:00 AM but unacceptable levels of contamination at 11:00 AM. Determination of frequency of tissue sampling must be statistically sound. A plant handling 1,000 cows a day will require more sampling than a plant handling

100 cows a day, but not necessarily 10 times more. Statistical tables (or a statistician) will usually need to be consulted.

d) A method for evaluating the effectiveness of the surveillance system must be determined. This will normally include an ongoing review of recorded data, particularly of the results of observations and testing at appropriate critical control points.

B. INVESTIGATION OF OUTBREAKS OF FOODBORNE DISEASE

Objectives

1. Describe the value of investigating outbreaks of foodborne disease as part of a total disease-control program.
2. Describe the procedures utilized in investigating outbreaks of foodborne disease and be able to apply them to a given problem.

Text

1. **Value of Investigating Outbreaks of Foodborne Disease.** Investigating outbreaks of foodborne disease involves applying principles of epidemiology to determine which food source was responsible for an outbreak and why.

Over the years, significant advances have been made in food technology to produce a wholesome product. Despite these advances, foodborne diseases remain important problems. In human medicine, reports of milk- and waterborne outbreaks have declined over the past 40 yr, but reports of foodborne outbreaks have remained fairly constant.

Investigation of foodborne outbreaks is an essential part of a total surveillance program. By accumulating data about outbreaks, three important objectives can be achieved. First, *controlling the disease* is made possible by the rapid identification of contaminated food sources, correcting faulty processing or preparation practices, and identifying and treating infected personnel. Second, *identification of etiologic agents* causing outbreaks is necessary. Cumulative data aid in making correlations among several outbreaks in which a causative agent was not identified to determine events common to all. With this information, probable etiologies can be proposed. In subsequent outbreaks, efforts can be made to increase the probability of identifying suspected agents. Third, *administrative guidance* based on valuable surveillance data can be offered. Various departments are thus better informed when attempting to implement disease-control programs.

Outbreak investigation often involves correlating disease data from several locales. When only a few individuals with rather mild symptoms are involved, the disease is often not regarded as foodborne. But when such information is reported to a single agency it can be examined for factors common to all outbreaks to determine the possibility of the disease being foodborne.

2. **Procedure for Investigating Outbreaks of Foodborne Disease**
   a) *Establishing the existence of an outbreak.* In human medicine the Centers for Disease Control (CDC) define an outbreak of foodborne disease as two or

more cases (except for botulism or chemical poisoning, for which one case constitutes an outbreak). That these cases result from a common source is understood. In veterinary medicine, a similarly precise definition does not exist. In addition, reporting is not adequate to regularly identify cases on multiple premises resulting from a common source. Therefore, it is easy to miss outbreaks.

b) *Verifying the diagnosis.* The first step in investigating an outbreak suspected of being foodborne is to verify the diagnosis. If the diagnosis is correct, it must then be decided whether the agent or circumstances are compatible with foodborne disease. The investigator looks for similarities among the patients' symptoms, signs, and incubation periods (time of onset of clinical illness) and attempts to identify any foods that all patients have recently consumed. With this information, it is possible to determine the probability that a foodborne outbreak exists.

The investigator is given a certain amount of information at the time a report is filed, but this is usually inadequate to determine the source of the causative agent. Also, some cases may not have been suspected of being foodborne at the time they were reported.

c) *Planning a detailed investigation.* Before the investigator conducts interviews and collects laboratory specimens, a detailed plan should be prepared that will give pertinent information.

d) *Organizing interviews or a survey.* Interviews with patients or clients are an important part of conducting an investigation. Appropriate questions can give important clues as to why some exposed individuals had signs and symptoms and others did not. On the other hand, poorly phrased questions can be misleading and produce erroneous answers. Responses to closed questions (those with "yes" or "no" answers) may often reflect patient or interviewer bias; an open question and a careful listener can gather more useful information. The first question that the investigator wants answered is, Where did the outbreak occur? A food can be contaminated through improper handling and/or unsanitary preparation, so the potential for food to become a source of a disease agent exists wherever food is processed, prepared, or served.

Certain foods have over the years been found to be associated more frequently with foodborne outbreaks. The investigator should watch for these potentially hazardous foods when reviewing attack-rate calculations.

Identification of the hazardous food results from the cooperative efforts of the investigator and the laboratory. The laboratory relies heavily on the investigator to identify foods likely to be involved. On the other hand, the laboratory's analyses of patients' specimens, as well as food samples, are important in identifying the agent and the source.

e) *Formulating a tentative hypothesis.* After the investigator has collected preliminary data about the circumstances surrounding an outbreak, a tentative hypothesis is formulated. For example, it may be suggested at this time that the agent is either infectious or noninfectious.

To accurately identify the source of the outbreak, the investigator should ask the following questions: (1) Is the agent responsible for the outbreak associated with a raw food source? (2) Did the outbreak occur because of faulty handling, processing, or preparation practices? (3) Was an improper environment maintained for holding the food(s) after preparation?

f) *Conducting an investigation*

1) *Unsafe sources.* One of the first questions that must be answered is whether the food was obtained from a source that may be unsafe. Sources of contamination of human foods include raw milk and milk products, shellfish from polluted waters, and cracked or checked eggs. Animal food sources include feed from a mill with a record of contamination, hay bailed in a field with a heavy stand of toxic plants, and contaminated carcass meats used in pet food.

Ingredients of a food product may be contaminated by improper storage practices. Storing chemicals such as pesticides near foods provides an excellent opportunity for contamination. Leaky pipes (especially sewer drains), insects, and rodents are also sources of contamination.

Many disease agents are spread by foods of animal origin. These may be infectious microorganisms or noninfectious agents. In the slaughtering process, they are transmitted readily to other carcasses when improper handling or contaminated equipment is used. Chemicals, either in the environment or iatrogenically introduced, also are found in foods of animal origin.

Some food products require use of uncooked ingredients. Food handlers should be advised not to use food from damaged containers, such as cracked eggs or dented cans. Numerous outbreaks have occurred following addition of cracked or checked eggs to milk in preparation of eggnog, hollandaise sauce, or ice cream.

2) *Faulty handling and preparation.* Foodborne outbreaks that occur as a result of unhygienic or improper food preparation can be attributed to either equipment or food handlers. In reality, the outbreak is always the result of human error, whether contamination is from equipment or worker.

In reviewing food preparation practices, the investigator should determine if the outbreak has been caused by cross-contamination during preparation. Raw foods of animal origin (poultry, eggs, and meat) are sources of bacteria in the kitchen. If the same utensils (knife, cutting board, etc.) are used for raw products and then later used for prepared foods without first being disinfected and cleaned, contamination is likely to occur.

Certain disease agents frequently are spread by personnel preparing foods. Enterotoxigenic staphylococci are spread most frequently by workers handling foods.

3) *Improper environment.* The factors needed for growth of microorganisms in prepared food before serving are (1) a sufficient nutrient (the *food* itself), (2) a proper environment for growth (*moisture* and *proper temperatures*), and (3) *time* for replication so that sufficient numbers are present to cause illness.

Some people, and especially food service establishments, routinely prepare food well in advance of when it is to be served. If the temperature at which the food is held is between 4.4°C (40°F) and 60°C (140°F), bacterial growth is encouraged.

Improper refrigeration is the factor associated most frequently with foodborne outbreaks. Therefore, the investigator should closely observe such practices.

g) *Analyzing the data*. After the investigator has conducted interviews, observed food handling areas and practices, and obtained laboratory results, the data can be analyzed to suggest a probable source of the agents that caused the outbreak. When several food items are involved it may be necessary to perform an *attack-rate analysis*.

To make this analysis, the interview data regarding consumption of foods and beverages obtained from individuals involved in an outbreak are summarized in tabular form. For each food, those who ate it and those who did not are tabulated. Each of these major categories is further subdivided into the numbers of those who became sick and those who did not.

Attack rates are then calculated for each food in relation to each group. (For an example, see Table 3.1).

To identify the food most likely to be the vehicle involved, the attack rate for persons eating each food is compared with that for persons not eating it, using the standard procedure for determining relative risk.

$$\text{Relative risk} = \frac{\text{Attack rate among those eating item}}{\text{Attack rate among those } not \text{ eating item}}$$

The food with the greatest relative risk is considered to be the food involved. In the sample attack rate table in Table 3.1, the greatest relative risk exists for those who ate the roast beef.

$$\text{Relative risk} = \frac{73.2}{8.3} = 8.82$$

Table 3.1. Sample attack-rate table

Food or Beverage	Persons Who Ate Specific Food				Persons Who Did Not Eat Specific Food			
	Sick	Not sick	Total	Attack-rate, %	Sick	Not sick	Total	Attack-rate %,
Roast beef	104	38	142	73.2	1	11	12	8.3
Potatoes, gravy	87	35	122	71.3	8	24	32	25.0
Green beans	76	30	106	71.7	25	30	55	45.4
Bread	55	20	75	73.3	50	45	95	52.6
Butter	55	20	75	73.3	50	45	95	52.6
Salad	3	7	10	30.0	98	57	155	63.2
Dessert	25	17	42	59.5	76	46	122	62.3
Coffee	60	40	100	60.0	39	21	60	65.0
Milk	13	7	20	65.0	85	55	140	60.7

h) *Testing the hypothesis.* After analyzing the data, the investigator must test the hypothesis. Analysis may be possible with available data (attack-rate calculations), or it may be necessary to conduct further laboratory tests or reexamine food-handling practices.

i) *Formulating a conclusion.* The investigator then attempts to assemble facts into a logical sequence to formulate a conclusion about factors that led to the outbreak.

j) *Implementing controls.* When a faulty step in the food chain is identified, it must be corrected. Often this is a matter of properly educating and supervising food handlers. If a specific food item is identified as the probable source of illness, further use of that food must be stopped until analyzed.

k) *Writing a report.* The final step in conducting an investigation involves writing a report. Disseminating reports of an outbreak is a valuable aid to other investigators who may at some time encounter a similar outbreak.

C. INSPECTION OF FOOD PRODUCTS

Objectives

1. Evolution of U.S. Federal Meat and Poultry Inspection
   a) Describe four methods by which meat and poultry inspection provides consumer protection.
   b) Describe four community benefits of meat and poultry inspection.
   c) Describe the historical development of current meat and poultry inspection laws.
   d) Compare the Wholesome Meat Act of 1967 with earlier meat inspection laws, emphasizing changes created by the act.
   e) Identify exemptions to the Wholesome Meat Act of 1967 and describe the significance of the Curtis Amendment.
   f) Compare the Wholesome Poultry Products Act of 1968 with earlier poultry inspection laws, emphasizing changes created by the act.
   g) Identify exemptions to the Wholesome Poultry Products Act of 1968.
   h) Describe why the Humane Slaughter Act of 1958 was developed and, given specific situations, be able to identify noncompliance.
   i) Describe and contrast the effectiveness, benefits, and disadvantages of humane stunning methods.

2. Evolution of Meat and Poultry Inspection in Canada
   a) Describe the historical development of current meat and poultry inspection laws.

3. Antemortem Inspection
   a) Define the following terms:
      1) Antemortem
      2) Suspect
      3) Condemned
      4) Subject to inspection
      5) 4D

6) Disposition
b) Describe why antemortem inspection is necessary.
c) Describe the antemortem inspection procedure and the equipment and facilities required.
d) Describe the types of dispositions that may be made of animals found to be abnormal on antemortem inspection.
e) Describe the dispositions and legal obligations associated with tuberculosis and brucellosis reactors and for animals suspected of having a reportable disease.

4. Postmortem Inspection
   a) Introduction
      1) Describe the general economic and food hygiene considerations involved in postmortem examination.
      2) Describe the reasoning behind the six basic food hygiene principles of postmortem examination.
      3) Define the following terms:
        (a) Condemned
        (b) Inedible
        (c) Denaturant
        (d) Decharacterize
        (e) Restricted
      4) Describe the procedures for the control of condemned and inedible material.
      5) Describe methods by which condemned or inedible products may be prevented from entering the human food chain.
      6) Identify conditions that make a carcass or product acceptable for animal food but not for human food.
   b) Infectious conditions
      1) Describe the three generalized conditions found at postmortem that will result in carcass condemnation.
      2) Describe several pathologic conditions resulting from microbial activity that are found commonly at postmortem and the criteria used in determining carcass disposition for each.
      3) Describe several pathologic conditions resulting from parasitism that are found commonly at postmortem and the criteria used in determining carcass disposition for each.
      4) Describe factors to be considered in decisions about the use of livers for human and animal food.
      5) Describe the basis for decisions regarding the disposition of various skin conditions, abscesses, and eosinophilic myositis.
   c) Noninfectious conditions
      1) Define emaciation and asphyxiation and describe the criteria for their condemnation.
      2) Describe the common pigmentary conditions that may lead to condemnation.
      3) Describe the conditions that are commonly involved in disposition of the liver.

      4)   Describe the more common neoplastic processes encountered in food-animal inspection and the criteria for their disposition.

      5)   Describe the criteria used for disposition of whole or parts of carcasses with the following conditions.

         (a) Bruises

         (b) PSE

         (c) Nephrosis

         (d) Chemical residues

         (e) Sexual odor

      6)   Explain conditions condemned for esthetic reasons, compared with those condemned as potential health hazards.

5.   Poultry Inspection

    a)   Describe the development of modern poultry inspection.

    b)   Describe the criteria for condemnation of the following avian conditions:

      1)   Tuberculosis

      2)   Leukosis

      3)   Septicemia-toxemia and synovitis

      4)   Cadaver

      5)   Contamination

      6)   Airsacculitis

    c)   Specify the temperature requirement for poultry that have reached a packaging area.

6.   Labeling and Shipping Meat and Meat Products

    a)   Describe the essential features of a label, including warning statements.

    b)   Describe how product labels should inform consumers of quality standards in production of meat and poultry products.

    c)   Describe inspection criteria for trucks used to ship meat or meat products.

    d)   Describe procedures followed when meat or meat products are returned to an abattoir.

    e)   Describe the Acceptance Quality Level program of inspection.

7.   Milk Inspection

    a)   List four potential health hazards that milk inspection prevents.

    b)   Inspection in the United States

      1)   Explain how the federal milk-marketing-order program influences the economy of the dairy industry.

      2)   Describe the PHS recommended standards for milk and milk products.

      3)   Describe the primary and the secondary responsibility for quality control of the dairy industry.

      4)   Define certified milk and describe some associated health hazards.

    c)   Inspection in Canada

      1)   Describe evolution of milk inspection in Canada.

Text

1.   Evolution of Federal Meat and Poultry Inspection in the United States

a) There are four major methods by which meat and poultry inspection provide consumer protection.

1) *Eliminating diseased meat.* The most important activity of an inspection program is preventing entry of diseased meat into the food chain. This is more effective than trying to separate unwholesome meat, poultry, or their products from wholesome products at the time of retailing.

2) *Esthetic factors.* Another reason for inspection is to prevent objectionable or undesirable meat from being sold to consumers. Consumer rejection on the basis of esthetics is a legitimate reason for not allowing certain meats to be marketed. Thus all meat that is rejected is not necessarily diseased.

3) *Clean equipment and environment.* Strict hygiene is essential to prevent foodborne infections and intoxications and provide high-quality meat and meat products for the consumer. Note that the objective here is prevention!

4) *Labeling.* Proper labeling is important to prevent adulteration and misrepresentation of products. Certain essential information must be included on the label, thereby providing consumers with criteria for evaluating the product. Proper labeling prevents processors from taking advantage of consumers.

b) *Benefits of meat and poultry inspection.* A good meat and poultry inspection program offers several benefits to the community.

1) *Statistical summary of the federal Food Safety and Inspection Service (FSIS).* Each year a statistical summary of all products from inspected meat plants provides a valuable aid to disease surveillance and control programs. The FSIS cooperates with other federal and state programs involved in disease control and eradication. An animal with tuberculosis, brucellosis, or taeniasis (cysticercosis) detected at slaughter, for example, is traced back to the farm of origin. Epidemiologic investigations can more precisely identify the source of infection.

The veterinarian in private practice who is advising food-animal-producing clients should be aware of the most common causes of condemnation. The summary data for antemortem and postmortem inspections for 1988 are shown in Tables 3.2, 3.3, and 3.4. In recent years the FSIS has ceased publishing separate summaries for antemortem and postmortem condemnations and currently provides only a summary of total condemnations, combining antemortem and postmortem results. The items indicated in Tables 3.2 and 3.3, therefore, are not precise for some conditions. If a condition can result in condemnation on either antemortem or postmortem inspection, the total number of animals condemned are listed under postmortem condemnation only. Many cows, for example, are condemned on antemortem inspection for epithelioma (cancer eye). However, since there is no reporting of antemortem inspection results separate from postmortem results and some condemnations for epitheliomas do occur as a result of postmortem inspection, all epitheliomas are listed under postmortem conditions.

2) *Prevention of disease.* Several disease agents may be transmitted through the food chain. Animal by-products from slaughtering are used in feed

for livestock as well as food for companion animals. Inspection helps to prevent transmission of these agents.

Table 3.2. Animals condemned on antemortem inspection for selected conditions, 1988

Conditions	Cattle	Calves	Sheep/Lambs	Goats	Swine	Equine
CNS disorders	273	144	34	8	300	3
Deads	9,548	16,021	3,483	622	59,852	85
Moribund	2,462	1,039	221	18	1,581	20
Pyrexia	412	20	19	1	179	2
Tetanus	15	2	1	0	11	1
Total	12,710	17,226	3,758	649	61,923	111
Total examined	32,790,091	2,437,383	4,801,694	235,408	79,128,870	300,263
Condemnation rate	.0004	.007	.0008	.003	.0008	.0004

Source: USDA, *Food Safety and Inspection Service Summary*, fiscal year 1988.
Note: Condemnation for these conditions was the result of only antemortem inspection. Conditions that resulted in some antemortem condemnations and some postmortem condemnations (e.g., epitheliomas) are not included.

Table 3.3. Animals condemned on postmortem inspection, 1988

Conditions	Cattle	Calves	Sheep/Lambs	Goats	Swine	Equine
Degenerative and dropsical conditions						
Emaciation	3,731	883	2,783	148	512	38
Miscellaneous degenerative conditions	3,964	55	32	12	796	14
Infectious diseases						
Actinomycosis, actinobacillosis	1,064	3	-	1	5	-
Coccidioidal granuloma	17	-	-	-	14	1
Swine erysipelas	-	-	-	-	2,780	-
Tuberculosis nonreactor	153	1	-	-	3,673	-
Tuberculosis reactor	15	7	-	-	-	-
Miscellaneous infectious diseases	141	14	30	-	145	7
Inflammatory diseases						
Arthritis	1,656	3,195	1,864	10	11,352	5
Eosinophilic myositis	3,105	12	182	-	8	-
Nephritis, pyelitis	3,513	188	143	3	2,053	7
Pericarditis	4,627	72	40	1	1,294	2
Peritonitis	6,314	1,361	92	18	7,732	40
Pneumonia	10,557	2,478	3,819	112	10,760	197
Uremia	1,063	26	749	7	846	4
Miscellaneous inflammatory diseases	2,486	425	42	2	765	15
Neoplasms						
Carcinoma	4,133	26	20	3	306	93
Epithelioma	18,134	3	-	-	10	4
Malignant lymphoma	13,413	98	86	1	1,191	19
Sarcoma	267	6	23	-	81	3
Miscellaneous neoplasms	474	14	11	5	1,048	75

Table 3.3. (continued)

Conditions	Cattle	Calves	Sheep/ Lambs	Goats	Swine	Equine
Parasitic conditions						
Cysticercosis	117	-	387	4	36	-
Myiasis	4	11	-	-	-	-
Miscellaneous parasitic conditions	201	1	1,525	7	249	-
Septic conditions						
Abscess, pyemia	10,874	503	736	75	23,303	40
Septicemia	12,207	2,766	536	27	8,223	91
Toxemia	5,346	632	478	57	3,275	43
Other						
Contamination	2,499	440	748	63	8,771	15
Icterus	639	5,036	885	19	8,072	6
Injuries	4,230	1,092	195	27	5,141	80
Pigmentary conditions	171	8	2	1	415	260
Residue	151	2,766	5	-	195	4
General miscellaneous conditions	275	62	28	-	4,650	5
Other reportable diseases	19	16	1	-	66	-
Mastitis	736	1	4	-	52	-
Metritis	1,679	-	6	-	302	-
Caseous lymphadenitis	-	-	4,547	181	-	-
Sexual odor	-	-	-	-	91	-
Total	117,978	22,201	19,996	784	108,203	1,069
Total examinations	32,790,091	2,437,383	4,801,694	235,408	79,128,870	300,263
Condemnation rate	0.0036	0.0039	0.0042	0.0033	0.0014	0.0036

Source: USDA, *Food Safety and Inspection Service Summary,* fiscal year 1988.
Note: In some instances, the figure represent combined antemortem and postmortem condemnation (e.g., epithelioma, abscesses).

Table 3.4. Food Safety and Inspection Service condemnation rates, by species, 1988

Conditions	Cattle	Calves	Sheep/Lambs	Goats	Swine	Equine
Condemnation	130,688	39,427	23,754	1,433	170,126	1,180
Inspected	32,790,091	2,437,383	4,801,694	235,408	79,128,870	300,263
Condemnation rate	.004	.016	.005	.006	.002	.004

Source: USDA, *Food Safety Inspection Service Summary,* fiscal year 1988.
Note: The figures represent combined antemortem and postmortem condemnation.

3) *Increased marketability of products.* Uniformity of meat inspection standards increases marketability by reducing trade barriers between localities caused by differences in criteria for an acceptable product. Federal standards for interstate shipment effectively eliminate local trade barriers.

4) *Consumer confidence.* Establishing consumer confidence that the product is wholesome is another important benefit of meat and poultry inspection.

c) *Beginnings of meat and poultry inspection.* The legal and esthetic bases for current meat and poultry inspection programs have evolved over many centuries, beginning in Egypt, where flesh from swine was considered unclean. By 200 B.C. the Jews had begun kosher slaughter. Antemortem and postmortem inspection began in Bavaria in 1615. France established a system of public abattoirs in 1807.

The first U.S. federal legislation on meat inspection was passed in 1890. The real basis for the current program, however, was the Meat Inspection Act of 1906. This act had strong support because some countries were refusing to import meat from the United States and public demand for legislation developed after exposes such as Upton Sinclair's *The Jungle*. The 1906 act provided for (1) antemortem and postmortem inspection of each animal; (2) prevention of diseased and unwholesome meat from entering food channels; (3) reinspection during processing; (4) continuous inspection; (5) truthful and informative labeling; (6) approval of floor plans and specifications; and (7) control of meat shipped interstate, imported from foreign countries, or sold to federal agencies. This program was administered by the Bureau of Animal Industry of the U.S. Department of Agriculture.

In the 1920s the USDA entered into agreements with certain state and local agencies to inspect poultry, either live or dressed. The federal Poultry Products Inspection Act was passed in 1957. Inspection extended to poultry under the 1957 act was similar to that already established for red meat in the 1906 act. The law provided for inspection of poultry in interstate commerce and from foreign sources.

d) *Wholesome Meat Act of 1967.* The purpose of the Wholesome Meat Act (WMA) of 1967 was to close loopholes in earlier laws that permitted sale of uninspected meat to the public. Its provisions are as follows:

1) *Inspection of all meat sold.* The first and most important of these changes was that all meat sold must be inspected, whether for sale in intrastate or interstate commerce or in export to foreign markets.

All meat for intrastate sale must be inspected in a program at least equal to the standards of the federal inspection act. Each state was required to develop such a program by December 1970. Compliance in the state was based on surveys of plants by federal and state inspection teams.

At the time the WMA was passed, 30 states had some form of mandatory antemortem and postmortem inspection, 13 states had voluntary inspection programs, 5 states had no statutes for inspection but did have some form of general food or sanitation laws for plants handling meat, and 2 states did not have inspection but had some form of licensing.

2) *Federal assistance to states.* A second important provision of the 1967 act was that a cooperative agreement could be developed between state and federal governments in which a state would be subsidized for up to half the cost of the state-operated program.

The state-federal agreement also could provide for federal assistance in training of inspectors, providing administrators to aid in supervision, training laboratory personnel, and sampling specimens for laboratory examination.

In spite of the federal subsidy provided, several states decided that they could not afford to carry on an inspection program for meat sold within the state under the requirements of the new law. The USDA does the inspection in these states and in states that have never had state programs.

3) *Designating plants as health hazards.* A third change included in the 1967 act gives the Secretary of Agriculture the authority to designate a plant a health hazard and close the plant. Plants handling dead, dying, diseased, or disabled animals can be closed to prevent such meat from reaching the public. Also, plants without potable water, proper sewage disposal, or adequate sanitation can be closed.

4) *Inspection of meat establishments in territories.* Another change required federal inspection of all meat-processing plants in the unorganized territories, such as Guam.

5) *Inspection of boner and cutter plants.* In the meat industry, plants referred to as *boners* and *cutters* receive whole carcasses and divide them into the primal cuts such as ribs, loin, shoulder, and round before further distribution in commercial channels. Before the 1967 act, plants receiving carcasses from federally inspected abattoirs could process and distribute the meat in interstate commerce as federally inspected on the basis of inspection in the previous plant. Now the several hundred boner and cutter plants that ship interstate must have federal inspection.

6) *Inspection of sausage-packing plants.* Before the 1967 act, plants that merely packaged sausage could apply for a certificate of exemption from federal inspection even though much of the product went interstate through catalog sales and sales to tourists. Now exemptions are no longer issued and not only must plants supplying products for interstate commerce be inspected but all their suppliers must be inspected as well. In practice, this has a domino effect, since each plant may have four or five suppliers.

7) *Authority over renderers, transporters, warehouses, and animal-food manufacturers.* The Secretary of Agriculture now has authority over plants rendering sick and dead animals into inedible products; transporters such as truckers, airlines and railroads; warehouses where meat may be stored; and manufacturers of food for animals such as pets, mink, and fish. The 1967 act required registration and periodic inspection of these plants, with an emphasis on preventing unwholesome meat from entering the food chain from any of these sources.

8) *Increased inspection of imported products.* Currently, the United States requires that a country wanting to ship a product here must meet three requirements: (1) its inspection law must be approved by the USDA as at least equal in stringency to the U.S. law; (2) its inspection procedures must be reviewed in person by a USDA veterinarian for compliance with the law; and (3) plants in the country must be approved individually. Australia, with the largest volume among approximately 40 countries supplying meat to the United States, has only a few of its plants approved. No country with endemic foot-and-mouth disease may ship

uncooked meat to the United States.

e) *Exemptions.* All loopholes were not eliminated. There were still two exemptions from inspection. First, custom plants that slaughter animals for the owner could be exempted. All the meat from these animals had to be returned to the owner for personal use. These plants were subject to sanitation and equipment inspections. Second, exemptions were allowed for retail dealers or stores that did not slaughter and at least 75 percent of whose sales were to retail customers. The retail store could cut up, slice, and trim carcasses into retail cuts; grind and freeze meat products; and even cure, smoke, and cook some products for retail customers only.

The Curtis amendment made an important change in the 1967 act. After passage of the act, it was recognized that there were many small custom plants that both slaughtered animals and had retail counters. To require inspection would force these operators to make expensive changes in their plants, so the act was amended to keep them in business on a legitimate basis. The custom operator must now stamp all custom-slaughtered meat "not for sale." All meat sold at the retail counter must be derived from inspected and passed carcasses (federal or state).

f) *Wholesome Poultry Products Act of 1968 (WPPA).* The USDA inspects all poultry in states that either never developed a state poultry inspection program or discontinued the state program after the act was passed in 1968. Federal inspection is a decided advantage in states such as Arkansas and Georgia, which have large broiler industries, and Minnesota, which has extensive turkey production, since most of these products enter interstate commerce.

The 1968 act permits two exemptions from inspection of poultry. The first allows farmers who raise up to 250 turkeys or 1000 chickens or combinations thereof annually to sell uninspected dressed birds directly to consumers, but not for resale.

The second exemption allows small processors to handle up to 5000 turkeys or 20,000 chickens/yr. The processing plant must still pass equipment and sanitation inspection, but each bird isn't inspected.

Poultry inspected under a state "equal to" program are not eligible for interstate commerce.

g) *Humane Slaughter Act of 1958.* The federal humane slaughter law, which became effective August 25, 1958, applied to all plants selling meat items to the federal government. Before 1958 a knocking hammer commonly was used to stun cattle. The effectiveness of this method depended entirely on the skill of the individual wielding the hammer. Although most cattle were stunned with the first blow, some required up to a dozen tries. Many times, especially with a novice handler, the aim would be inaccurate and an animal would be hit in the eye or on the side of the face. The Humane Methods of Slaughter Act of 1978 extended the law to include all federally inspected plants. The law regulates handling procedures in the abattoir up to and including the stunning process.

Hazards such as protruding nails are guarded against by the Humane Slaughter Act. There should be no obvious hazards for injury to animals in the abattoir, including holding areas.

Excitement of the animals must be kept to a minimum. Some people do not realize that driving animals with electric prods, chains, or boards with nails is inhumane. Animals should not be driven so that they climb over one another. Compassion is of utmost importance, and under this law, it is required.

The stunning area should provide good footing for the animal as well as limit its movement. It is important that stunning be complete before the shackles are attached to the animal. Hoisting and bleeding should be delayed until the animal is completely stunned.

h)   *Humane stunning methods*. Five methods of stunning are considered humane under the federal law.

1)   *Captive bolt guns*. When a captive bolt gun is discharged, a bolt protrudes from the gun. The bolt may be of two types, either a skull-penetrating type or a nonpenetrating (mushroom head) type. The disadvantage of the skull-penetrating bolt is that it passes through the hide and bone and enters the brain, thus contaminating it with normal skin flora.

2)   *Rifle with live ammunition*. Firearms are accepted as a humane method for stunning animals, but there is an important disadvantage to their use. Brain and head meat cannot be used for food because when the bullet hits the skull, it shatters and disperses fragments in many directions, thus contaminating tissues.

3)   *Electric stunning*. Electric shock is another accepted method for stunning animals. The electrical current and time are regulated to stun the animal and produce a state of anesthesia. Death occurs from subsequent bleeding produced by severing major arteries. An adverse effect is that excessive current may cause petechial hemorrhages in various organs. Since these hemorrhages also can indicate diseases such as hog cholera, an inspector then has the added difficulty of determining the cause. The "blood splash" from this method may be unacceptable to consumers, as well. In 1985, electric shock as a means of slaughter (as opposed to merely stunning) was approved. The procedure, referred to as *deep stunning* or *electrical slaughter,* is optional. With this technique, which uses a third electrode placed on the back or foot in addition to the two normally applied to the head, the "splashing" that accompanies electrical stunning is reduced. The weight of blood lost during bleedout appears to be identical to that achieved using other stunning methods.

4)   *Carbon dioxide*. The carbon dioxide (CO_2) chamber developed by Hormel and Company is used in some larger packing houses to produce surgical anesthesia in sheep, calves, or swine. The animals are shackled and bled as they come out of the chamber. CO_2 stunning is banned in some countries.

5)   *Kosher slaughter*. Ritualistic slaughter is approved by the Humane Slaughter Act. Kosher killing is done by hanging the animal and making a single instantaneous cut, severing the jugular veins and carotid arteries. The animal becomes unconscious from blood loss and dies. The killing is performed by a rabbi's assistant.

2. **Evolution of Meat and Poultry Inspection in Canada**
    The history of red meat and poultry inspection in Canada is similar to that in the
    United States but is complicated by the fact that the infrastructure of govern-
    ment changed dramatically in the same time period. In spite of this, inspection
    programs have been in place since the beginning of the nineteenth century.
    a) *Meat inspection.* The following is a time line of significant events:

    1805   The Upper and Lower Canada legislatures passed laws regulating
             the slaughter and processing of beef and pork.
    1800's   Certain municipalities began regulating the slaughter and processing
             of meat animals for human consumption.
    1850's   The Bureau of Agriculture came into existence (responsible for
             disease control in livestock and, eventually, meat inspection).
    1867   The British North America Act created a federal state in Canada,
             consisting of the provinces of New Brunswick, Nova Scotia, Ontario,
             and Quebec, and later including the ten Canadian provinces.
    1869   The Animal Disease Control Act was passed by the new federal
             government to regulate animal health.
    1873   Federal Beef and Pork Inspection legislation was passed.
    1907   The inauguration of the Inspection Service, which has become the
             Animal Inspection Directorate, was the Meat and Canned Foods
             Act passed in 1907. Inspectors were initially trained at the Chicago
             Veterinary College, but shortly thereafter, were trained in Canada.
             The Meat and Canned Foods Act regulated meat destined for
             interprovincial or export trade.

    b) *Poultry inspection.* Poultry inspection fell under the same federal legislation
        and jurisdiction as red meat at least as early as the first Canada Agricultural
        Products Standards (CAPS) Act, passed by Parliament in 1955, which in
        1980 became the Canada Agricultural Products Act, still known as CAPS.
            CAPS is a general act that controls inspection for wholesomeness and
        quality, and controls the marketing of agricultural products, which are
        defined under Chapter 27 of the Act as "an animal, plant, or an animal or
        plant product, or a product, including any food or drink, wholly or partly
        derived from an animal or plant." Because it also controls marketing, it sets
        the stage for supply management of agricultural commodities, specifically,
        dairy products and most poultry products, including eggs, broilers, turkeys
        and broiler chick production. Regulations are published and updated
        periodically for the implementation of the Act. The Meat Inspection Act,
        first adopted in 1955, elaborates and extends the provisions of the CAPS Act
        to red meat and poultry. It excludes caribou and other game species
        (important to indigenous northern peoples). The current meat inspection
        regulations are published to carry out in detail, the provisions of the Acts
        with regard to wholesomeness and safety of edible meat and poultry
        products.

3. **Antemortem Inspection**
    a) *Terminology.* The following terms are used in this presentation.

1) *Antemortem*. This term, which literally means *before death*, here refers to the inspection of an animal before it is slaughtered.

2) *Suspect animal*. This term refers to an animal possibly affected by a condition or disease that requires condemnation of the carcass, either wholly or in part, when slaughtered.

3) *Condemned animal*. This term refers to an animal that may not go to slaughter, judged as unfit for food at the antemortem inspection. The veterinarian bases the decision on clinical signs.

4) *Subject to inspection*. Occasionally, abattoirs establish conditions before purchasing an animal. In this situation the seller (the farmer) and the buyer (the packinghouse operator) agree on payment for that portion of the animal that passes inspection; thus the animal is purchased subject to passing inspection.

5) *4D*. This term is packinghouse jargon for animals that are dead, dying, diseased, or disabled.

6) *Disposition*. This term refers to the ultimate handling of a carcass, or its parts, after it has been inspected.

b) *Reasons for antemortem inspection*. There are several reasons for antemortem inspection. The most important is to remove from human food channels animals with conditions that cannot be detected at postmortem inspection. Several central nervous system (CNS) diseases, for example, manifest obvious clinical signs but cannot be readily detected at necropsy. Prior observation of the live animal is useful in making sound postmortem decisions.

Antemortem inspection also prevents unnecessary contamination of personnel and equipment inside the plant by diseased animals. This is very important from an economic point of view, as it avoids unnecessary plant shutdowns and cleanup.

Cooperative programs with other animal-disease-control agencies are an integral part of antemortem inspection. Many times the antemortem inspector is the first medically trained person to observe the animal clinically during its life. Therefore, the inspector is a vital link in many disease eradication programs.

Some animals that are clinically ill when received at the abattoir, and would probably be condemned on postmortem inspection, can be salvaged with proper treatment. If the abattoir management desires to treat a sick animal, the veterinary inspector can permit this, subject to certain controls. Swine erysipelas is an excellent example of a condition from which the animal might be salvaged, as it responds readily to antibiotic treatment.

c) *Antemortem inspection procedure*. It is imperative that antemortem inspection of animals be done on the day of slaughter. Some conditions are missed, even with this procedure. Nevertheless it is an effective method of discovering many animals unfit for food.

Antemortem inspection should include observations of the animal at rest and in motion. Lamenesses and locomotor abnormalities are best observed while the animal is walking or running. On the other hand, some physical abnormalities such as dyspnea and shivering are difficult to evaluate unless the animal is resting.

Based on a clinical evaluation, which may include temperature, pulse, and respiratory rate (TPR), the veterinarian decides whether the animal is normal.

Adequate facilities and equipment for antemortem inspection are important. Items needed include proper lighting, ventilation, drainage, and holding facilities. Restraining equipment must be well designed and constructed. Often the inspector may need to observe an animal closely to make an intelligent decision about the disposition.

Cleanliness is another important factor related to adequate antemortem inspection. If facilities are clean, animal discharges indicative of disease may be observed on the floor.

d) *Antemortem dispositions of abnormal animals.* Abnormal animals may be disposed of in three ways. (1) If the animal has a localized lesion that is not indicative of a generalized condition, it may go to slaughter. (2) Animals may be slaughtered as "suspects." A tag stating so is attached to the ear of these animals (or they may be tattooed) so that they can be identified in the abattoir. These animals are subject to postmortem inspection, at which time they may pass inspection, have a portion of the carcass rejected, or be condemned entirely. (3) If an animal is condemned in the plant, the carcass must be rerouted so that it does not enter the food channels. An animal that is condemned at antemortem inspection never enters the abattoir. Suspects are slaughtered last. (See Fig. 3.2.)

e) *Dispositions for commonly encountered conditions*
   1) *Scirrhous cords.* Swine with scirrhous cords may go to slaughter because the localized lesion and associated tissues will be rejected at postmortem inspection.

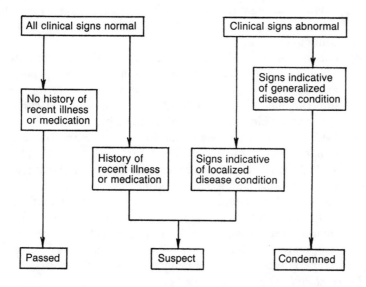

Fig. 3.2. Antemortem inspection and dispositions.

2) *Multiple abscesses.* In contrast, multiple abscesses usually indicate a generalized condition for which the animal must be condemned since it is unfit for food.

3) *Epithelioma.* Epithelioma (cancer eye) is seen commonly in Herefords. If the neoplasia is extensive and a secondary infection is present, or if the animal has become cachectic, condemnation is the logical disposition. On the other hand, if the tumor is less advanced, the animal may be tagged a suspect and sent to slaughter.

4) *Actinomycosis.* Actinomycosis (lumpy jaw) is an infectious disease caused by an anaerobic, non-acid-fast bacterium that forms abscesses in the mandibular region. Because this is usually a localized condition, the animal may be sent to slaughter as a suspect.

5) *Downer cow. Downer* animals (animals that are unable to stand or move about normally) present a complex problem. Any animal that fits this description may be withheld from slaughter for at least 24 hr. An exception to this is the animal that has had a traumatic injury during transport to the stockyard. In this instance, emergency antemortem inspection is appropriate since there is a good explanation for the animal's condition. In all other instances the 24-hr period allows the inspector time to observe for clinical signs. After 24 hr, if the animal's condition has worsened, it is condemned. If there is no change in the animal's health status, it may be slaughtered as a suspect. Samples are taken to determine if there are any tissue residues of drugs that might cause the downer condition.

6) *Pneumonia.* Dispositions of pneumonia cases vary. If the condition is advanced and generalized, the animal is usually condemned. In cases of lesser severity, the animal is sent to slaughter as a suspect.

7) *Central nervous system (CNS) damage.* There are several infections (e.g., listeriosis) that cause CNS damage and can be transmitted from food animals through the food chain to humans, in whom they produce similar lesions. Any animal with signs of current CNS infection is condemned.

8) *Retained placenta.* Animals that have recently given birth are fit for food. They are sent to slaughter as soon as the placenta has passed. Parturient animals used to be held 10 days before slaughter, but the belief that these animals are unfit for food has been abandoned with the realization that parturition is a normal physiologic process.

9) *Fever.* An animal is condemned at antemortem inspection if its body temperature is excessively high: for cattle, 40.6°C/105°F; for swine, 41.4°C/106°F). The veterinarian must take the ambient temperature into consideration. Animals can become overheated on hot days or with crowding, for example. In these situations, the animals may be cooled with water, moved to shaded areas, or provided a more favorable shelter, and reexamined later as suspects. Interestingly, minimum temperature guidelines have not been set; animals with subnormal body temperatures are *not* condemned solely on this basis.

f) *Reactors and reportable diseases*

1) *Tuberculosis reactors.* Tuberculosis (TB) reactors (which should be

identified by a T brand on the left cheek) are classified as suspects at antemortem inspection. The ear tag number and all antemortem findings are recorded to aid the postmortem inspector in making disposition judgments. Postmortem examinations are performed on any TB reactors that die in the holding pens. All information available about the animal is recorded and is extremely valuable to field investigation teams that are engaged in TB eradication.

2) *Brucellosis reactors*. It is interesting that bovine and porcine brucellosis reactors are simply identified by their ear tag number and then sent to slaughter. In other words, unlike TB reactors, they are not classified as suspects. The law states that brucellosis reactor goats are not to be slaughtered in an abattoir. Bovine brucellosis reactors are further identified by a B brand on the left cheek.

3) *Reportable diseases*. Whenever signs of anthrax, hog cholera, or vesicular disease are noticed, local state and federal livestock sanitary officials should be notified immediately. Authorities from these agencies will recommend to the inspector a disposition on the animal. These diseases are highly communicable; to avoid contamination of the entire area, the animals are held in isolation. The abattoir must not dispose of the animal before the appropriate agencies are notified because examination of it is an important link in animal disease control.

4. Postmortem Inspection
a) *Introduction*
1) *General considerations*. Reliable evidence and careful reasoning are essential to making proper disposition of a carcass at postmortem inspection. Unfortunately the guidelines for making the proper disposition often are not clear. Veterinarians must understand the effects that observed lesions may have on the wholesomeness of meat. Diseases of public health importance have been well described so guidelines related to them are quite clear. Consumers must be the first consideration when making a disposition of a carcass. Nutritional value and wholesomeness of the product are of prime concern. Esthetics is another important consideration. For example, wholesome meat may have unusual markings (e.g., those from hemorrhage) that may not appeal to consumers. Parenchymatous organs, such as the liver, spleen, or kidneys, must be examined for evidence of degenerative changes indicative of generalized disease processes. These changes may consist of enlargement or diminution in size, multiple hemorrhages or abscessation, or changes in normal color or consistency.

Veterinarians must prevent unnecessary wastage of the product when making a disposition. There must be a good reason for making a cut into an expensive piece of meat.

As the carcass is butchered, it is particularly important that the parts be accounted for. If an entire animal is to be condemned during postmortem inspection, a portion of it must not be allowed to enter commercial food channels.

Figs. 3.3 and 3.4 illustrate the decision-making procedures in postmortem inspections.

2) *Basic principles of postmortem disposition*

   (a) *Normal vs. abnormal tissue.* The first step is to separate normal from abnormal tissue as soon as possible. If the lesions are minor, such as bruises, they may be trimmed off without further consideration.

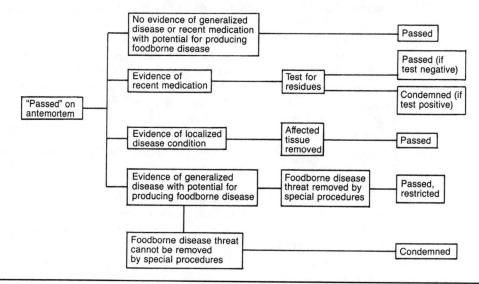

Fig. 3.3. Postmortem inspection and dispositions for animal "passed" on antemortem inspection.

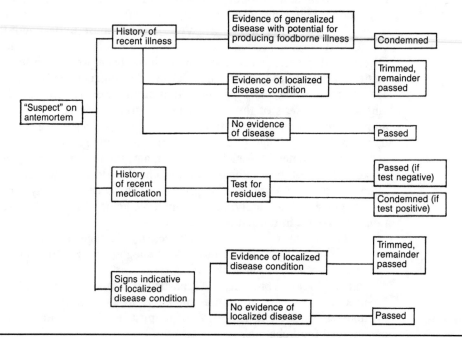

Fig. 3.4. Postmortem inspection and dispositions for animal evaluated as "suspect" on antemortem inspection.

(b) *Localized vs. generalized and acute vs. chronic conditions.* Next, determine whether the condition is localized or generalized and if it is acute or chronic. These conditions are essential in comprehending the pathologic process that may have resulted in a lesion. A well-encapsulated lesion is less hazardous than one that is active and spreading.

(c) *Conditions affecting physiologic functions.* Although the primary lesion may be localized, in some instances it may still have dramatic effects on other parts of the body. For example, a persistent urethral calculus will lead to uremia. Consequently, the animal must be condemned because of the generalized effect of the calculus on normal physiologic function.

Another example of a generalized condition that develops from a local lesion is seen in animals that become emaciated because of eating difficulty caused by excessively worn teeth.

(d) *Conditions injurious to consumer health.* On occasion, postmortem lesions may be difficult to recognize, yet a condition can exist that is hazardous to consumer health. Drug residues, for example, may pose an important threat to consumers.

(e) *Consumer acceptability.* Consumer acceptability is an important consideration that often determines whether or not a product can be passed for food. Some products cannot be used legally for food, whereas some may be used but usually are not because of consumer aversion. For example, bovine and hog tongues are used for food but most abattoirs will not market tongues from sheep and goats.

What is sold by the packinghouse, in the broadest sense, is determined by the market demand for the product, which in turn depends on cultural differences in particular areas. As a general rule, a product may be sold, assuming it has not been ruled illegal, if it is prepared in a hygienic manner. This standard is quite flexible. If a packer desires to salvage a product that is not usually marketed, a request may be sent to the central offices for meat and poultry inspection in Washington, D.C., for a ruling by a council of inspectors.

(f) *Product wholesomeness.* Finally, disposition of the product is based on its wholesomeness. Consumer acceptance is related to what the public regards as wholesome. For example, if the public is aware of unsanitary practices in abattoirs, the product most likely will not be accepted. In the United States, consumers expect animals to be slaughtered under sanitary conditions.

3) *Terminology.* The following terms are used in this presentation:

(a) *Condemned products.* These products are unwholesome because of disease or severe contamination.

(b) *Inedible products.* These products are unwholesome because they are not usually eaten and are not expected in food.

(c) *Denaturant.* This term refers to any substance that will change the appearance, taste, or smell of a product and will thus destroy the product for food purposes.

(d) *Decharacterize*. This term refers to changing the physical character (appearance) of a product in order to discourage its use as human food. Decharacterizing is used primarily for products that are condemned for human use but acceptable as ingredients of animal food. Approved green or red dyes can be used to decharacterize but are fairly expensive. Powdered charcoal is cheap, but it can be washed off.

(e) *Restricted products*. These are products that may not be sold without further processing, such as cooking or freezing.

4) *Control of condemned products*. Once a product has been condemned or deemed inedible at postmortem inspection, proper controls must be available to avoid subsequent mixing of these products with inedible products. Without this crucial step, all efforts to identify and separate inedible and condemned tissue from edible tissue are ineffective. Often, inedible and condemned products are very similar to edible products. Unless the former are removed immediately, it may be difficult later to identify any mixing. Since inedible and condemned products are both considered unfit for human consumption, they can be disposed of in the same way, by depositing them in a container marked inedible or condemned.

If the entire carcass or a cut is to be retained for further inspection or analysis, it is placed in a locked retained cage. Boxed or barreled meat also may be put in the cage. The key to this cage is retained by the inspector, and when the results of analysis are received, the inspector makes a disposition.

5) *Methods used to destroy inedible or condemned products*. The following four methods are used for destruction of inedible products:

(a) *Hashing*. The hashing and crushing process involves grinding bones, meat, blood vessels, fat, etc., preparatory to rendering. The ground material does not have the appearance of an edible product. This procedure must be done in areas of the plant that are segregated from edible-product processing.

(b) *Rendering*. *Rendering* (melting down) is a method that is practical only in high-volume plants.

(c) *Incineration*. Although incineration is an acceptable method for disposal of inedible and condemned products, it seldom is used because of cost and air pollution.

(d) *Denaturing*. Application of a denaturing agent is the most common method of destroying these products. This is done by pouring or sprinkling the agent on the product. If the agent is applied to products in a barrel, it should be done in layers so that it is well dispersed throughout the barrel. Large cuts of meat and carcasses should be cut into or slashed before applying the agent. Cresylic disinfectant is one of the most commonly used denaturants because it is available in most plants (used for disinfecting trucks and premises).

6) *Animal food*. Several conditions encountered in postmortem inspection require that the entire carcass be condemned for use as human food

although it may still be acceptable for use in animal food: for example, anasarca, emaciation, eosinophilic myositis, immaturity, nonseptic bruises, epithelioma, sarcosporidiosis, and unborn calves.

Products intended for use in animal food must be handled so that they are separated from edible food products to avoid subsequent mixing.

Some condemned livers can be used for animal foods. Conditions such as telangiectasis, "sawdust" liver, and livers with parasitic scars are acceptable. They must be slashed and decharacterized first.

b) *Postmortem disposition of infectious conditions.* The conditions described herein are those most frequently encountered at postmortem inspection in the abattoir. In examining a carcass, the veterinarian must remember that the lymph nodes are key indicators of infection or neoplasia in the areas drained by them. A lymph node that is abnormally large, hemorrhagic, or abscessed should act as a red flag to the individual doing the postmortem.

1) *Generalized infectious conditions.* There are three generalized conditions that may be encountered at postmortem inspection.

(a) *Septicemia.* Septicemia is a generalized disease; the lesions vary but often are characterized by congestion, hyperemia, petechial hemorrhages, tissue edema, lymphadenopathy, or interference with normal blood clotting. Often these are indications of degenerative changes that are occurring in parenchymatous organs, such as the liver, kidney, and spleen. Inspection of these organs is essential during postmortem examination. In this instance, the carcass is condemned because it is a potential health hazard and is esthetically unacceptable to consumers.

(b) *Pyemia.* Pyemia is generalized abscessation. The animal may have concurrent septicemia, but in such situations the presence of pyogenic organisms can be demonstrated. In addition to generalized abscesses, there may be hemorrhages involving the kidneys and/or lymph nodes. Lesions similar to septicemia may be noted in parenchymatous organs. The carcass must be condemned.

(c) *Toxemia.* Toxemia results from systemic absorption of toxins that are produced originally at a local site of infection. The systemic changes, which are similar to those with pyemia and septicemia, also result in carcass condemnation.

2) *Pathologic conditions of bacterial and/or viral etiology.* There are several conditions of microbial etiology that require sound judgment when making a disposition at postmortem examination.

(a) *Tuberculosis.* Although tuberculosis (TB) is relatively infrequent now, it is still important because it has not been eradicated and poses a public health threat.

TB is a granulomatous, inflammatory disease. Because of the predilection of the agent for lymphoid tissue, lymph nodes are examined routinely at postmortem inspection. TB in cattle is particularly a disease of the respiratory system.

Infection with mycobacteria in swine, however, is usually of the avian type associated with the gastrointestinal system and does not produce classic tubercles. It is important for farmers to segregate chickens from swine. Avian TB may be transmitted to hogs either by bird droppings or as a result of eating dead birds.

The carcass of a tuberculous animal can be passed for food without restrictions in a few instances. If the lesions are confined to a single system in swine, the carcass may pass; for example, if only mesenteric and cervical lymph nodes are involved, the gastrointestinal system may be discarded and the remainder used for food. This might be regarded as an intermediate category. If the carcass is passed restricted, it must be stamped and the meat cooked at a standardized time and temperature (76.7°C/170°F for 30 min). Cattle that are TB-test-negative and free from lesions are passed unrestricted; cattle that are TB reactors and free from lesions are passed only for cooking.

There are several circumstances in which cattle or swine carcasses must be condemned when lesions are noted at postmortem inspection: generalized lesions, antemortem pyrexia, cachexia; lesions in muscle, bone, joint, or abdominal organ; lesions extensive in thoracic or abdominal cavity; and lesions that are multiple and active.

In federally inspected plants, special effort is made to identify tuberculous cattle. Granulomatous lesions found during postmortem examination of TB-reactor cattle are collected and sent to the National Animal Disease Center in Ames, Iowa, for etiologic identification. In the plant, all lymph nodes from these animals are incised and examined and the hide is spread out and examined for lesions.

(b) *Arthritis*. Arthritis often is of bacterial etiology. At postmortem examination, enlarged joints and occasional congestion and hyperemia of an associated lymph node are seen. Change in synovial fluid may be noted grossly. Arthritis and polyarthritis often are observed in animals at postmortem but are not reasons for condemnation unless associated systemic changes are present.

(c) *Pneumonia*. Although not all causes of pneumonia are infectious, a significant proportion are. Pneumonia varies from a single focus of infection to extensive involvement, the degree of which is important in determining carcass disposition. The stage of pneumonia influences the decision. For example, a gray cast to the lung parenchyma indicates massive leukocytic infiltration, which may represent a progressive disease process or convalescence. Therefore, the veterinarian must rely on associated signs in making an intelligent disposition. In this instance, antemortem inspection is important.

Mediastinal lymph nodes and pleura are important indicators of the condition of the respiratory system. The gross appearance and extent of involvement of these structures aid in determining if a respiratory disease is localized or systemic.

(d) *Pericarditis*. Pericarditis frequently is caused by infectious organisms.

The condition is encountered most often in cattle. The extent varies from a localized lesion to extensive systemic involvement. Disposition of the carcass depends on extent of involvement, that is, whether the condition is localized or generalized, acute or chronic, and active or inactive. Investigation to determine possible sites of secondary infection is important.

(e) *Actinobacillosis.* Actinobacillosis and actinomycosis are handled similarly to pericarditis. It must be determined if there is systemic involvement; if not, the affected part may be excised.

(f) *Caseous lymphadenitis.* Caseous lymphadenitis frequently is encountered in the slaughter of sheep. Depending on degree of involvement, the affected part may be excised or the entire carcass condemned.

3) *Pathologic conditions of parasitic etiology.* Several parasitic conditions may be encountered when examining a carcass at postmortem. The veterinarian should categorize the degree of involvement as (1) generalized, (2) local organ involvement with systemic manifestations, or (3) simply localized infection.

(a) *Bovine taeniasis.* Bovine taeniasis (cysticercosis, beef measles) is caused by the intermediate stage of the tapeworm *Taenia saginata.* Humans, the definitive host for the parasite, contract the infection by eating meat of infected cattle. Special attention is given at postmortem to the heart and masseter muscles, because these tissues are infected most frequently. Occasionally, the diaphragm is examined. Postmortem disposition depends on the degree of tissue involvement.

Carcasses that are not extensively involved may be treated by excising apparent cysts and holding continuously at $-26.1°C$ ($-15°F$) for 15 days. It is essential that the 15-day time be continuous. The cysts are destroyed when the meat is heated to $60°C$ ($140°F$), but this means of control cannot be regulated as effectively as freezing.

(b) *Swine taeniasis.* Humans are the definitive host for pork taeniasis and, more important, can also be the intermediate host. Therefore, this disease agent is of major concern. Disposition of carcasses affected with this disease is not the same as that for beef measles. *Any* lesion of taeniasis (*Cysticercus cellulosae*) requires at least a "passed restricted" disposition. Excessive infestation calls for condemnation of the carcass.

(c) *Swine ascariasis.* Normally, swine ascarids are a localized condition. Occasionally, ascarids occlude the common bile duct, thus precipitating obstructive jaundice. With this systemic involvement, the animal must be condemned. Ascarids migrate through the liver during their development within the host and produce fibrous scars. The liver is edible, but the scars or tags must be removed first.

(d) *Tongue worms.* The parasite *Gongylonema pulchrum* inhabits the submucosa of the tongue of swine. Postmortem examination involves palpating the tongue to search for the parasite and to detect abscesses. In some instances, large tongues must be split and each half palpated. If abnormalities are not detected, the tongue is passed for food after scalding.

(e) *Trichinosis*. Trichinosis has been a major concern of consumers for many years. Primarily through effective public education, its occurrence has declined steadily in the United States. This disease in swine is not detected readily at postmortem inspection. Continued decline in occurrence of human cases will depend primarily on successful education of the public to cook all pork thoroughly. Cooking of garbage for swine feeding (required by law) and application of newer testing methods have reduced the prevalence of trichinae in swine.

For control purposes, all pork is assumed to be infected. Proper preparation of pork in the kitchen is relied on for effective control, except for pork products with a ready-to-eat appearance. In the latter products, one of four methods is utilized to destroy the trichinae: heating, freezing, salting and drying, or irradiation.

(1) *Heating*. Pork must be heated to a temperature of 55°C (131°F) to kill trichinae. Meat plants are required to heat the meat to 58.3°C (137°F), which allows a safety margin, or to use a combination of temperature and holding time proven to destroy trichinae.

(2) *Freezing*. The freezing temperature varies with the product and its salt content, but instant freezing to −40°C (−40°F) in the center of the meat is used in plants to kill trichinae for some ready-to-eat products that will probably not be reheated.

(3) *Salting and drying*. Salting and drying are used primarily on products such as dry sausage. Drying by itself is not a reliable means of destroying trichinae. However, in the presence of salt, the cyst becomes dehydrated by osmosis.

(4) *Irradiation*. A dose level between 20 and 30 Krad prevents the maturation of encysted larvae in meat.

(5) *Pooled sample detection of trichinae*. The pooled sample technique for trichinosis control must be done correctly to ensure success. First, sampling and analysis must be done rapidly before hogs are cut up and parts dispersed. Second, all incoming hogs must be identified so that trichina-positive animals can be traced to the farm of origin. The pooled sample technique involves pooling diaphragm samples from groups of 20 to 25 hogs, digesting the muscle, and examining the pooled samples microscopically for cysts. If the sample is positive, a second muscle sample is obtained from each hog and run separately to identify the infected individuals.

4) *Liver*

(a) *Abscess*. Approximately 10 percent of the cattle inspected in the United States have abscessed livers. Any abscessed liver is condemned for human food but some can be trimmed and used in animal food.

(b) *Fluke damage*. Flukes also account for condemnation of many livers.

In the United States any evidence of fluke infestation renders the liver unfit for human consumption. In other countries, however, flukes may be trimmed out and the liver passed for food. Some flukes (*Dicrocoelium* sp.) are transmitted by ingestion of raw liver, which is done in certain cultures. Because of the public health importance of flukes, infected livers should be condemned. In the United States these livers usually are condemned for esthetic reasons only, because most liver is cooked before eating.

(c) *Parasitic scars*. Scars caused by migrating parasites other than flukes are seen commonly in livers of sheep, swine, and cattle. The livers may be used for human food after the scars have been trimmed out.

5) *Skin conditions, abscesses, and eosinophilic myositis*

    (a) *Skin conditions*. Many skin conditions, some of which are infectious, are handled as local lesions and simply trimmed out. If there are associated systemic changes, the whole carcass is condemned.

    (b) *Abscesses*. Abscesses usually are localized and may be trimmed out. Care must be taken when excising abscesses to prevent carcass contamination. Exudate from an abscess should not be washed off, as rinsing simply disseminates the pus.

    (c) *Eosinophilic myositis*. Eosinophilic myositis, a condition usually found in young, well-fattened cattle, is of uncertain etiology. It is discussed along with infectious conditions because there are many indications that this disease may be infectious. Lesions appear as yellowish green, spindle-shaped foci in the muscle fiber and may (grossly) be mistaken for sarcosporidiosis lesions. Postmortem examination and disposition of affected meat is similar to that used for bovine cysticercosis.

c) *Postmortem disposition of noninfectious conditions*

1) *Emaciation and asphyxia*. Two generalized physiologic conditions are encountered at postmortem inspection: emaciation and asphyxiation (or suffocation).

    (a) *Emaciation*. Although emaciation is frequently suspected at antemortem inspection, it cannot be determined definitely until postmortem. It must be differentiated from cachexia and mere leanness. *Cachexia* is associated with chronic debilitating diseases and is diagnosed more often during antemortem inspection. On the other hand, *emaciation* results from either inadequate caloric intake (starvation) or increased caloric demand as a result of stresses such as cold weather; otherwise the emaciated animal is essentially normal. In either emaciation or cachexia there is serous infiltration, or mucoid degeneration, of adipose tissue. A lean animal does not have this pathologic change and is normal and healthy with a minimum of fat stores. Emaciated animals are esthetically unacceptable for food.

    (b) *Asphyxiation*. *Asphyxiation* (suffocation) is indicated when the tissues are engorged with blood. It results from improper sticking, after stunning, with subsequent inadequate bleeding. This condition is seen most commonly in hogs that drown in the scalding tank before hair removal. These animals are considered unsound and are, therefore, not accepted for food. Several lesions, such as petechial hemorrhages, may be masked by the retention of blood.

2) *Pigmentary conditions.* Three pigmentary conditions are encountered at postmortem: icterus, melanosis, and xanthosis. Pigments are produced either endogenously or exogenously.

(a) *Icterus. Icterus* is increased bilirubin in the body as a result of a pathologic state in the hepatic or hemic systems. The affected animal is condemned. Icterus must be differentiated from similar-appearing conditions associated with diet or breed characteristics, such as seen in Jersey and Guernsey cattle. To detect icterus, tissues are examined that should normally be white, such as the intima of large vessels, sclera, tendons, connective tissue, pleura, and joint surfaces. These tissues, which are usually white even in breeds with yellow fat, will have a distinct yellow color if the animal is icteric.

(b) *Melanosis. Melanosis* refers either to an abnormal increase in or to an aberrant location of melanin deposits. Melanin pigment is found normally in the skin, brain, tongue, and palate. If melanin deposits found elsewhere can be trimmed out, the carcass can be saved. This condition must be differentiated from *melanoma,* a neoplastic condition.

(c) *Xanthosis. Xanthosis,* which develops from accumulation of waste pigments (lipochromes) in skeletal and cardiac muscles, is more common in older animals. In rare instances xanthosis is so extensive that the carcass must be condemned, but usually affected muscles can be trimmed and the remainder of the carcass used for food.

3) *Liver*

(a) *Cirrhosis.* There are many causes of cirrhosis of the liver, most noninfectious. These livers may be used for animal food but *not* human food. This condition is determined easily by cutting through the tough and fibrotic tissue.

(b) *"Sawdust" liver.* This is a term used in meat inspection for livers with characteristic small white or yellow necrotic spots on the surface. They are seen often in young, well-fattened cattle. The etiology of this condition is uncertain, but it is thought to be related to telangiectasis or abscesses. However, many sawdust foci never become abscessed. At present, if the foci are slight, they may be removed and the remaining liver used for food.

(c) *Telangiectasis. Telangiectasis,* a dilation of blood vessels, is a condition affecting beef livers. Telangiectasis often is seen on the surface as red spots that extend into the parenchyma. With aging, the spots become somewhat larger, darker, and more indented. Disposition of a telangiectic liver is similar to that of sawdust liver.

4) *Neoplasia*

(a) *Embryonal nephroma.* Embryonal nephroma is a tumor commonly seen in swine. It usually is well circumscribed and benign. Unless secondary changes are present, it is handled as a localized lesion and the carcass is passed for food after trimming. This tumor is seen less frequently in other species.

(b) *Malignant lymphoma.* No matter how slight the extent, a carcass with malignant lymphoma must be condemned. Usually involvement is generalized and the animal debilitated, so recognition is not difficult. Involved lymph nodes have a claylike consistency with red streaks throughout.

(c) *Epithelioma.* Epithelioma or squamous cell carcinoma (sometimes called *cancer eye*), a common eye tumor seen primarily in cattle, must be differentiated from other ocular conditions such as traumatic injury or a corneal dermoid. Animals with this condition may be consigned to slaughter subject to postmortem inspection when special attention is given to the parotid lymph nodes. This tumor usually metastasizes via the parotid node to the atlantal and thoracic lymph nodes. Any extensions of this tumor beyond the eye is reason for carcass condemnation.

5) *Miscellaneous noninfectious conditions.* Several noninfectious conditions are encountered commonly at postmortem examination.

(a) *Bruises.* Bruises are the result of traumatic injury with subsequent trapping of blood in and around muscle bundles and associated structures.

Shortly after the injury, the regional lymph nodes begin to swell and become darkened. Bruised tissue may be trimmed out and the remaining normal tissue used for food.

(b) *Pale soft exudative (PSE) pork.* PSE pork involves the muscle. The meat is considered wholesome and can be used as food. Occasionally a slight odor is present, which can be detected after chilling the carcass for 24 hr.

(c) *Nephrosis.* In nephrosis, depending on the duration and severity of the lesions, several systemic changes may occur. As severity increases, uremia becomes more pronounced. If there are secondary changes in the liver, spleen, etc., the condition is advanced and the animal is unfit for food. If fat from a uremic animal is heated, it will emit a urinelike odor. Uremia may exist in the presence of only minimal gross lesions.

(d) *Chemical residues.* Chemical residues are important. Most residues are not obvious at postmortem examination. If an animal is suspected at postmortem of containing residues (either from an evident injection site or suggestive history), the carcass is put in the retained cage for subsequent laboratory analysis. Legal tolerance levels and withdrawal times are revised periodically, and it is the veterinarian's responsibility to be acquainted with current regulations.

(e) *Sexual odor.* An offensive odor may be emitted when meat from adult male swine (boars, stags, or cryptorchids) is cooked. Those that produce a strong sexual odor cannot be passed for food but may, however, be incorporated in a comminuted product such as sausage (passed restricted). Boar meat often is sent directly to the rendering facility.

(f) *Immaturity.* Meat from animals slaughtered at a very young age is usually pale in color and friable as a result of a higher water content than that found in meat from mature animals. Meat from calves slaughtered during the first 3 weeks of life (150 lb or less) is called *bob veal.*

6) *Condemnation basis of common noninfectious conditions.* Although the meat and poultry inspection program has done much to improve uniformity of inspection throughout the United States, the basis for dispositions may be obscure to those not involved in the program. In 1968, the amendment to the WPPA stated that condemnations must be based on scientific facts or criteria. Nevertheless, most commonly encountered noninfectious conditions are condemned for esthetic reasons, that is, if a condition is offensive, even though not a hazard to human health.

5. **Poultry Inspection**

a) *Chronology of poultry inspection.* Nationwide mandatory poultry inspection is relatively new. Not until 1957 were laws passed requiring poultry meat in interstate commerce to be inspected for wholesomeness. A major stimulus for mandatory poultry inspection was the vast increase in size of the poultry meat industry, starting in the 1940s. Starting in the late 1920s "voluntary" inspection for wholesomeness was done by some packers, forced on them by regulations of various large city health departments that prohibited sales of uninspected poultry. Elsewhere poultry was still sold as live birds to be killed and inspected by the homemaker, restaurant cook, or butcher, or was marketed as "New York dressed" poultry (a trade term for a bird that has had only its feathers and blood removed, sold with all the viscera, including the digestive tract and its contents). Since 1968, inspection has been required for practically all poultry.

b) *Conditions resulting in carcass condemnation*

1) *Avian tuberculosis.* The occurrence of tuberculosis is almost always in older fowl, predominantly those from the north central states. Although it occurs in all states, the north central states have more small farm flocks that are slaughtered in commercial slaughterhouses. *Mycobacterium avium* can infect mammals, including humans, swine, sheep, mink, and rabbits. Tuberculosis lesions in poultry are characterized by central caseation but are *not calcified.* Affected carcasses are condemned.

2) *Leukosis (lymphoid).* Lymphoid tumors in chickens usually are caused by one of two common viral agents: Marek's disease virus or the lymphoid leukosis virus group. The lesions may resemble those of tuberculosis, with tumors in the bone marrow, liver, and spleen.

With Marek's disease, changes such as irregularities in diameter of the vagus nerve usually are easily detectable. Ovarian tumors are another lesion commonly seen in Marek's disease. Male birds often have testicular involvement with diffuse or nodular enlargement. Marek's disease also is manifested by changes in the feather follicles; only a few follicles may be affected or nearly the whole skin.

Lymphoid leukosis virus may produce bony changes. A carcass with evidence of leukosis is condemned.

3) *Septicemia-toxemia and synovitis.* Infectious diseases other than tuberculosis and the leukosis complex usually are classified as septicemia-toxemia or as synovitis. Any evidence of systemic involvement is reason for condemnation, since there is danger of transmitting infection to persons eating the meat. Signs of systemic involvement are (1) dehydration, (2) color changes (of skin, liver and other parts), (3) hemorrhages, (4) swelling of the liver (edges rounded rather than sharp), (5) swelling of the spleen, and (6) necrotic areas. Any one of these signs alone may not be sufficient for condemnation.

In synovitis the joints may have a collection of thick, almost gelatinous exudate tinged with blood. A purulent or caseous material may be found in some joints. Causes of the condition include species of *Mycoplasma, Staphylococcus, Salmonella,* and *Pasteurella.* Carcasses with synovitis are condemned.

4) *Cadavers.* A *cadaver* is a bird that died from causes other than normal slaughter procedures. Lack of bleedout is the criterion, and such a bird is condemned.

5) *Contamination.* A carcass may be condemned for contamination if, for example, the skin was torn by the picking machine, which would allow nonpotable water from the scald vat or picking machine to get under the skin.

6) *Airsacculitis.* This is an infection involving the air sacs. A severe case may be accompanied by pericarditis, perihepatitis, and peritonitis.

c) *High carcass temperature.* Regulations call for the temperature in a carcass that has reached the packing area to be 4.4°C (40°F) or less. This is one of the many requirements designed to prevent microbial growth.

6. **Labeling and Shipping of Meat and Meat Products**
   a) *Essential features of a label.* The label must contain five pieces of information: product name, ingredients, firm's name and address, net weight statement, and inspection legend. If any part of the label is missing or incomplete, it cannot be approved.
   1) *Product names.* The product name must be the common name that would occur normally on the product or that fully describes it. This is important, for example, if buying luncheon meat. There is an important difference between sliced ham and ham loaf!
   2) *Ingredients.* The ingredient statement must include *all* the ingredients included in the product. When more than one ingredient is used, the label must list them in order of decreasing predominance.
   3) *Firm's name and address.* A complete address, including zip code, must be included on the label. But it may not be the place where a particular product was produced; instead, it may be the name and address of a firm for whom the product is manufactured or of the general offices.
   4) *Net weight.* The federal Meat and Poultry Regulations explicitly state the form in which net weight is indicated on a label. Depending on the stated label weight, the requirements are as follows: (1) less than 1 lb, in ounces; (2) 1 lb but less than 4 lb, in ounces and also in pounds and

a fraction or the decimal equivalent (e.g., 20 oz and also 1 ¼ lb *or* 20 oz and 1.25 lb); (3) 4 lb and over, in pounds and a fraction or the decimal equivalent (e.g., 5 ½ lb *or* 5.5 lb).

5) *Inspection legend.* The inspection legend is included in the label on all federally inspected processed and packaged meat. A number in the legend is assigned to the establishment at which the meat was inspected and is unique to it. The poultry inspection label is different in that the lettering is bolder than that used for meat and the letter "P" precedes the establishment number. The legend is circular for poultry and red meat. Only federally inspected meat may have this form. The legend for state-inspected meat and poultry must be an alternative form, such as an outline of the state.

6) *Other information as required.* A warning statement, such as "Keep under refrigeration," may be required on the label if the product has not been thermally processed to be commercially sterile. Such items are found in retail store, self-service, refrigerated display cases. Canned hams that are heated only to an internal temperature of 65.6°C/150°F are not sterile, so the warning indicates that the product must be refrigerated. Statements for heated smoked pork products (not canned) such as "cooked," "fully cooked," or "ready to eat" imply that the products have been heated to a temperature of 64.4°C (148°F) and have a cooked appearance, that is, the meat has a cooked color and separates easily from the bone.

b) *Labeling and quality standards.* Improper labeling, whether intentional or accidental, can mislead consumers about product quantity or quality. The following are examples of misleading labeling.

1) *Origin of the product.* It is important to indicate the origin of a product. Products originally unique to an area but currently manufactured elsewhere, such as Italian, Swedish, or New England sausage must have the origin on the label. A product label with a term indicating a geographic significance is permissible provided the geographic term is qualified by a word such as *style, type,* or *brand* in the same size and style lettering as the geographic term.

2) *Quality of the product.* A label should not misrepresent quality, as in instances in which imperfect bacon slices from ends and pieces are represented as a quality product.

3) *Quantity of product.* If a product weighs between 1 and 4 lb, the label must represent the quantity with a dual declaration such as 20 oz (1 lb 4 oz). People are generally impressed with larger numbers and thus might be misled.

4) *Nutritive value of the product.* Generally, bacon contains relatively little red meat, which is the primary source of protein in the product. The statement "high in protein" is misleading, primarily because an established standard currently is not available to classify protein levels.

5) *Color of the label.* Red lines in a transparent bacon wrapper make the label unacceptable because they make the product appear leaner than it actually is. Also, the transparent window must reveal the major portion of the length of a representative slice.

6) *Proper filling.* Proper container filling is important to avoid misrepresentation. For example, if a jar contains Vienna-style sausages tightly packed against the wall, while the center is either empty or loosely filled, it may appear to contain more sausages than it actually does.

7) *Composition of the product.* Meat and poultry inspection regulations establish specific standards for each product produced in plants under federal inspection. For example, *ground beef* (or chopped beef) must consist of chopped fresh and/or frozen beef *without* the addition of beef fat and must not contain more than 30 percent fat. *Hamburger* must consist of chopped fresh and/or frozen beef *with or without* the addition of beef fat and must not contain more than 30 percent fat. The 30 percent fat for ground beef or hamburger established a standard of consumer expectancy.

c) *Shipping.* Shipping, the final link in bringing food to retailers, is as important as processing to ensure consumers a wholesome product. It does little good to enforce rigorous controls for processing if the product can become contaminated in transit to retailers. Before loading, trucks should be examined for cleanliness of floors, walls, top hooks, and roof. If necessary, they should be washed and cleaned completely. If there are holes or protruding wood or metal, the truck should not be used, as these conditions increase the probability of product contamination.

If the truck is in acceptable condition, the product should be loaded in a manner that minimizes possibility of contamination. Products should be examined for proper labeling. When carcasses are shipped, they should be hung from the overhead rail rather than laid on top of each other because hanging carcasses are contaminated less easily during transit. Drain holes in the truck, also a possible means of contamination, must be plugged before the product enters. Carcass meat nearly always is boxed before shipment nowadays, thereby reducing contamination.

d) *Returned products.* Some products are returned to the abattoir by dissatisfied purchasers. Before their reentry into the plant, an inspector examines the products for wholesomeness. If the inspector cannot examine a product immediately, it is placed temporarily in a retained cage.

e) *Acceptable quality level program.* The federal meat inspection program has developed an alternate procedure for examining carcasses. Because inspectors have found it virtually impossible to perform critical inspection of every carcass after it leaves the kill floor, the Acceptable Quality Level (AQL) program was developed.

In this program, carcasses are grouped in lots. Inspectors select sample carcasses at random and examine them very closely. Wholesomeness of the lot is determined by findings in this sample. For example, if inspectors observe a few hairs on a carcass, it would be termed a minor defect. Nevertheless, the processor would have to reroute this lot of carcasses for subsequent trimming. A more serious defect, such as evidence of malignant lymphoma, would be termed critical. In this instance, the whole lot would have to be reinspected with tighter controls to determine disposition.

7. Milk Inspection in the United States

a) *Principal milk inspection objective.* The principal objective of milk inspection is to safeguard human health from four major hazards: *milkborne infection, antibiotic contamination, toxic chemicals,* and *hazardous radionuclides.* To meet this objective, there must be continuous surveillance of the product from the farm through retail sale.

   Although the principal objective of milk inspection is to protect human health from milkborne hazards, the consumers, distributors, and producers derive important additional benefits. Recognition of the safety of milk fosters consumer acceptance of this relatively inexpensive nutritional source. Distributors benefit economically from increased shelf life resulting from the high sanitary standards required for production and processing.

b) *Milk marketing.* The dairy industry is probably the most regulated of all food industries, with regulation taking many forms. Milk market orders are an economic control, establishing the price that processors must pay dairy farmers for milk. The federal milk-marketing-order program is administered by the USDA.

   Federal milk-marketing areas fix the price on approximately 90 percent of total fluid milk and milk products consumed in the United States. Marketing orders are established at the request of dairy farmers. A formula is used to set a minimum price that is believed to be most equitable for farmers.

   In addition to economic regulations, there are sanitary regulations that have been (and in some areas still are) artificial trade barriers. Within the United States there are 20,000 state, county (or parish), and local (or municipal) health and sanitation jurisdictions. Plants processing milk for fluid consumption within these jurisdictions are inspected an average of 24 times/yr (in one state the average was 85), whereas the PHS milk ordinance recommends, as of April 1975, once every 3 mo. This excessive number of inspections occurs when more than one agency is involved in an inspection program and has cost milk producers, processors, and distributors more than $1 million/yr in excess of the tax funds used to support these duplicate programs.

c) *PHS standards for milk.* The PHS milk ordinance provides chemical, bacteriologic, and temperature standards as well as sanitation requirements for production and processing of Grade A raw and pasteurized milk and milk products. Some processors may offer monetary incentives for producers to meet more stringent standards to improve milk quality.

   1) *Standards: Grade A raw milk for pasteurization.* Grade A raw milk for pasteurization must be cooled to 7.2°C (45°F) within 2 hr after milking and maintained at that temperature or less until it is processed; milk from an individual producer cannot have more than 100,000 bacteria/ml, or after commingling with milk from other producers, not more than 300,000 bacteria/ml before pasteurization. There can be no detectable antibiotic residues.

   2) *Standards: Grade A pasteurized milk and milk products.* The standards for Grade A milk after it has been pasteurized require that the milk be cooled to 7.2°C (45°F) or less and maintained at that temperature. There can be no more than 20,000 total bacteria/ml with no more than

10 coliform bacteria/ml, and the phosphatase test must be negative.

3) *Standards: Grade A pasteurized cultured products.* For Grade A pasteurized cultured products such as buttermilk or cottage cheese, there is no limit on the total bacterial count but the coliform count must remain less than 10/ml. The temperature and phosphatase requirements are the same as for pasteurized milk.

d) *Responsibility for quality control of milk.* Primary responsibility for control of milk quality within a state rests with the state. A state agency, usually the health department, administers the program. In many states, actual inspection may be performed by personnel in a local agency, usually the health department or department of agriculture. This function has been delegated to the local agency by the state, which retains primary responsibility.

e) *Certified milk.* The American Association of Medical Milk Commissions was a nongovernmental organization that did much to improve the quality of fluid milk sold by establishing high standards for production of certified milk. Dairymen could adhere to these standards voluntarily and, in return, market their product labeled *Certified.* The program emphasized pure, clean, *raw* milk. In spite of the high standards, lack of pasteurization has resulted in some milkborne disease outbreaks from certified milk. These have been associated especially with *Salmonella dublin,* a strain of *Salmonella* that localizes in the cow's udder and is shed in milk, and *Campylobacter jejuni.*

8. **Milk Inspection in Canada**
   a) *Overview.* Milk inspection in Canada is a joint federal/provincial responsibility. The federal act governing milk quality, the Canada Product Standards Act, sets the minimum standards to which provincial regulations must conform. Standards set for milk are similar to those put forth in the PHS milk ordinance in the United States.
   b) *Milk marketing.* The Canadian dairy industry has been a supply managed system since the early 1970s, with federal jurisdiction over trade between provinces and foreign trade, and has created two markets for milk in Canada: the industrial market, which is federally regulated, and the fluid market, which is provincial. The Canadian Milk Supply Management Committee, which has representation from producers and governments in all provinces except Newfoundland, sets a national production target, which is adjusted periodically to reflect changes in demand. Each province allocates its share of the national quota to its producers according to its own policies. The target price for industrial milk is the level of return efficient milk producers should receive to cover cost of milk production and is based on an annual survey of 350 farms in Ontario, Quebec, and New Brunswick.

   Each province has the responsibility for meeting the table milk and fresh cream requirements of its own residents. By convention (not by contract or written agreement), fluid milk products in one province are not shipped to another province. There is no interprovincial competition in fluid milk products. The authority to market milk is delegated by provincial governments primarily through milk marketing boards financed and managed by producers. The degree of government control varies by province. Provinces establish price levels for fluid milk in a manner similar to the federal government for industrial milk. Provincial agencies may set fluid milk prices at the producer, wholesale, or retail levels, and in some instances, at all three levels.

The purpose of supply management is to provide a balance between the supply of raw milk and the demand of for milk and milk products at the national level. The Canadian market is primarily supplied by Canadian production, except for a few cheeses and other products not available from domestic sources. Because of this, Canada has a wide range of measures to monitor and control imports of dairy products.

c) *Responsibility for quality control of milk.* Provincial departments of agriculture carry out milk testing programs at the farm level. Standard tests at the farm level detect unsafe bacteria levels (Standard Plate Count, Plate Loop Test), presence of added water, and inhibitors. Specific provinces do additional testing to address regional concerns. For example, British Columbia tests for pesticide residues in milk. In most instances, milk quality affects the price producers get for their milk through a penalty system. Provincial inspectors also monitor products for quality and safety in processing plants that do not ship out of province. On-site inspection of the farm is part of the provincial inspection process. The frequency of inspection and testing differ from province to province.

Processing plants for industrial milk (destined for powder, butter, cheese, etc.) that ship out of province are also federally registered and inspected. This falls under the mandate of Agriculture Canada's Food Inspection Directorate. In Ontario and Quebec, provincial inspectors conduct federal inspections, subject to federal audit. In other provinces, there is cooperation between federal and provincial inspectors, especially if there is a particular problem in a plant. Inspections in the plant, in addition to checking for coliforms, also check for toxins (e.g., pesticides and herbicides) in the product.

Testing at retail level is undertaken by Consumer and Corporate Affairs in Canada, in conjunction with Health and Welfare Canada and Agriculture Canada. Testing is done randomly to verify product composition. Some provinces also monitor products on the retail shelf.

d) *Certified milk.* There is no federal provision for the testing and marketing of raw milk. It is discouraged in Canada.

D. BIBLIOGRAPHY

1. Preventing Foodborne Disease

Ayres, J. C., F. R. Blood, C. O. Chichester, H. D. Graham, R. S. McCutcheon, J. J. Powers, B. S. Schweigert, A. D. Stevens, and G. Sweig (eds.). 1968. *The Safety of Foods: An International Symposium.* Westport, Conn.: AVI Publishing.

Booth, N. H., and A. B. Holt. 1975. Toxicologic significance of drug and chemical residues. Proc. 20th World Vet. Congr. 1:203-7.

Charm, S. E. 1978. *The Fundamentals of Food Engineering.* 3d ed. Westport, Conn.: AVI Publishing.

_____. 1978. There is a new 15 minute test for penicillin in milk. *Hoard's Dairyman*

123:1034-35.

Engel, R. E. 1977. Nitrites, nitrosamines, and meat. *J. Am. Vet. Med. Assoc.* 171:1157-60.

Epley, R. J., P. B. Addis, C. F. Allen, and J. C. Worthesen. 1975. *Nitrite in Meat.* Anim. Sci. Fact Sheet No. 28. St. Paul: Agricultural Extension Service, University of Minnesota.

Federal Register. Feb. 1, 1972. *Use of Antibiotics in Animal Feeds.* Washington, D.C.: U.S. Government Printing Office.

Graham-Rack, B., and R. Binstead. 1973. *Hygiene in Food Manufacturing and Handling.* 2d ed. London: Food Trade Press.

Gunther, F. A., and J. D. Gunther (eds.). *Residues Rev.* 63(1976) to date. New York: Springer-Verlag.

Guthrie, R. K. (ed.). 1988. *Food Sanitation.* 3d ed. Westport, Conn.: AVI Publishing.

Heid, J. L., and M. A. Joslyn (eds.). 1967. *Fundamentals of Food Processing Operations: Ingredients, Methods, and Packaging.* Westport, Conn.: AVI Publishing.

Kimball, D. R. 1977. Public health regulations in milk quality control. *J. Am. Vet. Med. Assoc.* 170:1212-13.

Kramer, A., and B. A. Twigg. 1973. *Quality Control for the Food Industry.* 3d ed. Vol. 1, *Fundamentals* (1970); Vol. 2, *Applications.* Westport, Conn.: AVI Publishing.

Longree, K. 1980. *Quantity Food Sanitation.* 3d ed. New York: Wiley-Interscience.

_____. 1982. *Sanitary Techniques in Food Science.* 2d ed. New York: Macmillan.

Mercer, H. D. 1981. Prevention and management of drug and chemical residues in meat and milk. *In Current Veterinary Therapy*, ed. J. L. Howard, pp. 388-93. Philadelphia; W. B. Saunders.

Peterson, M. S., and D. K. Tressler (eds.). 1963/1965. *Food Technology the World Over:* Vol. 1, *Europe, Canada and the United States, Australia:* Vol. 2, *South America, Africa and the Middle East, Asia.* Westport, Conn.: AVI Publishing.

Potter, N. N. 1986. *Food Science.* 4th ed. Westport, Conn.: AVI Publishing.

Price, C. D. 1977. Monitoring for inhibitors and adulterants. *J. Am. Vet. Med. Assoc.* 170:1210-11.

Schell, O. 1984. *Modern Meat.* New York: Random House.

Sinclair, U. 1906. *The Jungle.* Reprint. New York: New American Library, 1961.

Smith. L. L. W., and L. J. Minor (eds.). 1974. *Food Service Science.* Westport, Conn.: AVI Publishing.

Stallones, R. A., chairman. 1980. *The Effects on Human Health of Subtherapeutic Use of Antimicrobials in Animal Feeds.* Washington, D.C.: National Academy of Sciences.

Swann, M. M. 1969. *Joint Committee on the Use of Antibiotics in Animal Husbandry and Veterinary Medicine: Report.* London: Her Majesty's Stationary Office.

Thorner, M. E. 1973. *Convenience and Fast Food Handbook.* Westport, Conn.: AVI Publishing.

U.S. Congress. Office of Technology Assessment F-91. 1979. *Drugs in Livestock Feed.* Vol. 1, *Technical Report.* Washington, D.C.: U.S. Government Printing Office.

_____. Office of Technology Assessment F-103. 1979. *Environmental Contaminants in Food.* Washington, D.C.: U.S Government Printing Office.

_____. Senate. Committee on Agriculture, Nutrition, and Forestry. 1979. *Food Safety. Where Are We?* Washington, D.C.: U.S. Government Printing Office.

U.S. Department of Health, Education, and Welfare. Food and Drug Administration. 1975. *Monitoring Drug Use in Animals.* DHEW/FDA Publ. No. 76-3006. Washington, D.C.: U.S. Government Printing Office.

2. Investigation of Outbreaks of Foodborne Disease

Bryan, F. L. 1973. *Guide for Investigating Foodborne Disease Outbreaks and Analyzing Surveillance Data.* Atlanta, Ga.: Center for Disease Control.

Greenberg, A. E., M. D. Taras, R. D. Hoak, and M. C. Rand (eds.). 1985. *Standard Methods for the Examination of Water and Wastewater.* 16th ed. Washington, D.C.: American Public Health Association.

Hendricks, S. L., chairman. 1966. *Procedure for the Investigation of Foodborne Disease Outbreaks.* 2d ed. Shelbyville, Ind.: International Association of Milk, Food, and Environmental Sanitarians.

Latham, R. H., and C. A. Schable. 1982. Foodborne hepatitis at a family reunion. Use of IGM-specific hepatitis A serologic testing. *Am. J. Epidemiol.* 115(5):640-45.

Mann, J. M., C. L. Hatheway, and T. M. Gardiner. 1982. Laboratory diagnosis in a large outbreak of type A botulism: Confirmation of the value of copraexamination. *Am. J. Epidemiol.* 115(4):598-605.

O'Mahoney, M., P. L. Clark, N. D. Noah, and H. E. Tillett. 1983. A foodborne outbreak of gastroenteritis of unknown aetiology. *Community Med.* 5(1):54-58.

Palmer, S. R., and B. Rowe. 1983. Investigation of outbreaks of salmonella in hospitals. *Br. Med. J.* 287(6396):891-93.

Pan American Health Organization. 1982. *Sanitary Control of Food.* Sci. Publ. No. 421. Washington, D.C.: World Health Organization.

Reimann, J., and F. L. Bryan (eds.). 1979. *Foodborne Infections and Intoxications.* 2d ed. New York: Academic Press.

Richardson, G. H. (ed.). 1985. *Standard Methods for the Examination of Dairy Products.* 15th ed. Washington, D.C.: American Public Health Association.

Shiffman, M. A., chairman. 1974. *Foodborne Disease: Methods of Sampling and Examination in Surveillance Programmes.* WHO Tech. Rep. Ser. No. 543. Geneva: World Health Organization.

Speck, M. L. (ed.). 1984. *Compendium of Methods for the Microbiological Examination of Foods.* Washington, D.C.: American Public Health Association. U.S. Department of Health, Education, and Welfare. Public Health Service. 1978. *Grade "A" Pasteurized Milk Ordinance:* Recommendations to the United States Public Health Service, Food and Drug Administration. PHS Publ. No. 229. Washington, D.C.: U.S. Government Printing Office.

U.S. Department of Health and Human Services. 1984. *Proceedings Second National Conference for Food Protection,* May 9-11, 1984. Washington, D.C.: U.S. Government Printing Office.

Watson, R. N., M. F. Stringer, R. J. Gilbert, and D. E. Mahoney. 1982. The potential of bacteriocin typing in the study of *Clostridium perfringens* food poisoning. *J. Clin. Pathol.* 35(12):1361-65.

3. Inspection of Food Products

Agriculture Canada. 1983. *Meat Hygiene Manual.* Ottawa, Ontario: Agriculture Canada, Food Protection and Inspection Branch.

Amstutz, H. E. (ed.). 1980. *Bovine Medicine and Surgery.* 2d ed. 2 vols. Santa Barbara, CA.: American Veterinary Publications.

Association of Medical Milk Commissions. 1972. *Methods and Standards for the Production of Certified Milk.* Association of Medical Milk Commissions, Inc., 2266 No. Prospect Ave., Suite 514, Milwaukee, Wis. 53202.

Blood, D. C., J. A. Henderson, and O. M. Radostits. 1983. *Veterinary Medicine.* 6th ed. Philadelphia: Lea & Febiger.

Canada Agricultural Products Act. 1988. Chapter 27. Ottawa, Ontario.

Canada Agricultural Products Standards Act. 1979. *Dairy Products Regulations. Canada Gazette Part II,* vol. 113:4260-4314. Ottawa, Ontario.

Canada Dairy Commission. 1989. *The Canadian Dairy Industry.* Ottawa, Ontario.

Cole, H. H., and M. Ronning (eds.). 1980. *Animal Agriculture: The Biology of Domestic*

Animals and Their Use by Man. 2d ed. San Francisco: W. H. Freeman.

Doull, J., C. D. Klaasen, and M. O. Amdur. (eds.). 1980. *Casarett and Doull's Toxicology: The Basic Science of Poisons.* New York: Macmillan.

Dunn, A. M. 1978. *Veterinary Helminthology.* 2d ed. London: William Heinemann Medical Books.

Fowler, S. H. 1961. *The Marketing of Livestock and Meat.* 2d ed. Danville, Ill.: Interstate.

Fraser, C. M. (ed.) 1986. *Merck Veterinary Manual.* 6th ed. Rahway, N.J.: Merck.

Griffiths, H. J. 1978. *A Handbook of Veterinary Parasitology.* Minneapolis: University of Minnesota Press.

Haagsma, N., A. Ruiter, and P. B. Czedik-Eysenberg (eds.). 1990. *Proceedings of EuroResidue Conference on Residues of Veterinary Drugs in Food.* University of Utrecht, Netherlands: Faculty of Veterinary Medicine.

Hofstad, M. S., B. W. Calnek, C. F. Helmboldt, W. M. Reid, and H. W. Yoder, Jr. (eds.). 1984 *Diseases of Poultry.* 8th ed. Ames: Iowa State University Press.

Jensen, R. 1982. *Diseases of Sheep.* 2d ed. Philadelphia: Lea & Febiger.

Jensen, R., and D. R. Mackey. 1979. *Diseases of Feedlot Cattle.* 3d ed. Philadelphia: Lea & Febiger.

Jones, T. C., and R. D. Hunt. 1983. *Veterinary Pathology.* 5th ed. Philadelphia: Lea & Febiger.

Jubb, K. V. F., and P. C. Kennedy. 1984. *Pathology of Domestic Animals.* 3d ed. 2 vols. New York: Academic Press.

Kon, S. K. 1975. *Milk and Milk Products in Human Nutrition.* 2d rev. ed. FAO Nutr. Stud. No. 27. Rome: Food and Agriculture Organization.

Kramer, A. 1973. *Food and the Consumer.* Westport, Conn.: AVI Publishing.

Lawrie, R. A. 1968. *Meat Science.* 3d ed. New York: Pergamon Press.

Lawrie, R. A. (ed.). 1980, 1981, 1985. *Developments in Meat Science.* Vols. 1-3. Amsterdam: Elsevier.

Laws of Prince Edward Island. 1987. *Dairy Industry Act.* Charlottetown, P.E.I.

_____. 1988. *Dairy Industry Act. Regulations.* Charlottetown, P.E.I.

Leman, A. D. (ed.). 1986. *Diseases of Swine.* 6th ed. Ames: Iowa State University Press.

Levie, A. 1970. *The Meat Handbook.* 3d ed. Westport, Conn.: AVI Publishing.

Levine, N. D. 1980. *Nematode Parasites of Domestic Animals and of Man.* 2d ed. Minneapolis, Minn.: Burgess Publishing.

Libby, J. A. (ed.). 1975. *Meat Hygiene.* 4th ed. Philadelphia: Lea & Febiger.

Mann, I. 1960. *Meat Handling in Underdeveloped Countries.* Rome: Food and Agriculture Organization.

Merchant, I. A., and R. A. Packer (eds.). 1967. *Veterinary Bacteriology and Virology.* 7th ed. Ames: Iowa State University Press.

National Research Council. Commission on Life Sciences Food and Nutrition Board. 1985. *Meat and Poultry Inspection. The Scientific Basis of the Nation's Program.* Washington, D.C.: National Academy Press.

_____. 1987. *Poultry Inspection, The Basis for a Risk-Assessment Approach.* Washington, D.C.: National Academy Press.

Price, J. F., and B. S. Schweigert (eds.). 1971. *The Science of Meat and Meat Products.* 2d ed. San Franscisco: W. H. Freeman.

Sloss, M. W., and R. L. Kemp. 1978. *Veterinary Clinical Parasitology.* 5th ed. Ames: Iowa State University Press.

Soulsby, E. J. L. 1982. *Helminths, Arthropods and Protozoa of Domesticated Animals.* 7th ed. Baltimore: Williams & Wilkins.

Thomson, R. G. 1984. *General Veterinary Pathology.* 2d ed. Philadelphia: W. B. Saunders.

Timony, J. F. 1988. *Hagan and Bruner's Microbiology and Infectious Diseases of Domestic Animals.* 8th ed. Ithaca, N.Y.: Cornell University Press.

3-A Sanitary Standards Committee. Sanitation in Dairy Equipment. In *3-A Sanitary Standards*. 3-A Sanitary Standards Committee, 5530 Wisconsin Ave., Washington, D.C. 20015.

United Nations. Food and Agriculture Organization. 1970. *Joint FAO/WHO Expert Committee on Milk Hygiene, Third Report*. FAO Agric. Stud. No. 83. Rome: Food and Agriculture Organization.

U.S. Department of Agriculture. 1968. *The Federal Milk Marketing Order Program*. USDA Agric. Mark. Bull. No. 27 (Apr.). Washington, D.C.: U.S. Government Printing Office.

U.S. Department of Health and Human Sciences. 1969. *Dairy Inspection and Grading Services*. USDA Agric. Mark. Bull. No. 48. Washington, D.C.: U.S. Government Printing Office.

_____. Animal and Plant Health Inspection Service, Meat and Poultry Inspection Program. 1979. *Meat and Poultry Inspection Regulations*. Washington, D.C.

_____. 1988. *Dollars and Sense, Proceedings of the Symposium on Animal Drug Use*. DHHS Publ. No. (FDA) 88-6045. Washington, D.C.: U.S. Government Printing Office.

Wiggins, G. S., and A. Wilson. 1976. *Color Atlas of Meat and Poultry Inspection*. New York: Van Nostrand Reinhold.

INDEX